VEGAN STRONG

VEGAN STRONG

THE ULTIMATE FIELD MANUAL
FOR A KICK-ASS PLANT-FUELED LIFE

SGT Vegan AKA Bill Muir, RN, BSN

SGT Vegan Press

2018

SGT Vegan Press
Los Angeles, California
www.sgtvegan.com

ISBN 13: 978-1719406901
ISBN 10: 1719406901

Library of Congress Control Number: 2018906271

Cover Design by William Brunet
Interior Design by Greg Gubi
Edited by Shawna Kenney
Interior Illustrations by David Wentworth
All Photos by the author, unless noted otherwise

Printed in the United States of America

DEDICATION

First and foremost, this book is dedicated to my
Mom, for her assistance with this project. It's
also dedicated to animal and human rights
crusaders, and to the worldwide vegan
movement. And finally, a shout out to our
brothers and sisters in the armed services.
Freedom isn't free.

CONTENTS

PART 3
VEGAN DELICIOUS

PART 4
VEGAN PEOPLE

ACKNOWLEDGEMENTS

Thanks to everyone who allowed me to use their stories in the book. Thank you to those who read the initial drafts and gave me feedback, especially Lisa Sanchez and Sarah Burns from the Veterans Writing Project, J. Curtis Strickland, and my siblings, Amanda Muir and Luke Muir. Thanks to my Mom for all of the countless hours of editing and encouragement. Finally, thank you to Ian MacKaye for his thoughts on the Punk Rock Chapter and for helping me to get an "Edge" on life.

INTRO

VEGAN: A person who does not eat any food that comes from animals and does not use animal products.

– The Merriam-Webster Dictionary.

VEGAN STRONG. My belief that being vegan not only promotes physical health and strength, but also makes us mentally and spiritually badass.

– SGT Vegan

LADIES AND GENTLEMEN in Reading Land, good day to you! Welcome to *VEGAN STRONG*! I am SGT Vegan (that's short for "Sergeant") and I am going to present a unique perspective to the vegan discussion.

I started my vegan journey in 1992. Since then, I've had a rather diverse resume: marathon runner, US Army Paratrooper, Combat Medic, Martial Arts Instructor in Southeast Asia, world traveler. I even managed to sing on the soundtrack of *Fantasy X,* widely considered one of the greatest video games of all time. Now I work as a Registered Nurse at the West Los Angeles VA Medical Center, where we fight against the lifestyle diseases plaguing our nation's veterans. Being an RN isn't a career -- it's a calling. As I have been vegan all over the world – through jungles, deserts, forests, combat zones (AND family vacations) – I feel called to share this knowledge with you.

VEGAN STRONG is divided into four parts. Part One discusses what it means to be vegan. Part Two touches upon nutrition and exercise. In Part Three, we'll learn some easy-to-make vegan dishes (being vegan doesn't have to be a mystical undertaking). And in the fourth and final part, there are interviews with vegans from different career fields, from all walks of life.

Being vegan is **easy** and **essential** to the survival of the planet. After reading this you'll be able to "vegan" with the best of them. Welcome to the next generation of vegan. Welcome to *VEGAN STRONG!*

Part 1

VEGAN STRONG

Chapter 1

Why Vegan?

WHY DO PEOPLE CHOOSE TO BE VEGAN? There are obvious reasons, such as superhuman strength, immortality, X-ray vision, and the ability to fly (SGT VEGAN NOTE: Some results may vary). The main reasons most people go vegan are for their health, for the environment, and because of compassion towards animals.

HEALTH

Let's start with health. Some people may believe that going vegan for your health is a selfish move. However, concern for your health and taking positive action to improve it is one of the best things you can do for yourself. Many of our society's health problems would be eliminated if we were to embrace a plant-based diet. If Americans adhered to a vegan diet, we would be freed from ailments that are plaguing our society, such as heart disease and diabetes. According to the *Epic-Oxford Study* published in 2013, vegans have a 32% lower risk of coronary artery disease than meat eaters. They also have lower Body Mass Index, lower LDL and blood pressure[1]. When meat eaters say that something is missing from the vegan diet, they're correct; it's the cholesterol and fat present in all animal products, which are what is causing obesity and heart attacks!

People who eat less animal products are living longer and looking better. This isn't just my opinion; it's science. Doctors have been taking their sweet time getting around to it, but now they will agree that a vegan diet (also called a "plant-based diet") can be as healthy or even healthier than the Standard American Diet (SGT VEGAN NOTE: Please check out Physicians Committee for Responsible Medicine – www.pcrm.org for information from a group of doctors who are promoting a vegan diet).

The American Dietetic Association recently stated that appropriately planned vegan diets are healthful, nutritionally adequate, and may provide health benefits in the prevention and treatment of certain diseases. Well-planned vegan diets are healthy for individuals during all stages of the life cycle, including pregnancy, lactation, infancy, adolescence, and adulthood. The results of an evidence-based review showed being vegan is associated with a lower risk of death from ischemic heart disease. Vegans also appear to have lower low-density lipoprotein cholesterol (LDL) levels, lower blood pressure, and lower rates of hypertension and Type 2 diabetes than non-vegans. Furthermore, vegans tend to have a lower body mass index and lower overall cancer rates. Features of a vegan diet that may reduce risk of chronic disease include lower intakes of saturated fat and cholesterol and higher intakes of fruits, vegetables, whole grains, nuts, soy products, fiber, and phytochemicals.[2]

Eating meat negatively impacts:

1. Your Brain. Autopsies of Alzheimer's patients have shown their brains had an unusual amount of cholesterol.[3] Yes, your body needs cholesterol; it is a vital component of your biology. That's why your body produces all the cholesterol you need. Dietary cholesterol is ONLY found in animal-sourced foods. The extra cholesterol you get when you CHOOSE to eat animals hardens your arteries in a process

called arteriosclerosis, eventually cutting off the circulation of blood to the places you need it most, like your heart and brain. Let's think about this for a minute. No blood going to your heart? Bam! You get a heart attack. No blood going to your brain? Bam! You have a stroke. Remember, dietary cholesterol is only present in animal based foods, and you can choose to lower your cholesterol overnight by eliminating your dietary cholesterol consumption.

2. <u>Your Heart</u>. Vegans have a 32% lower risk of coronary artery disease than meat eaters.[4] I don't want you to miss this point; dietary cholesterol is the leading cause of heart disease. The cholesterol you are eating is choking your arteries, and hurting your ticker.[5] Western Medicine would have you take potentially harmful pills to lower your cholesterol. How about just not eating the extra cholesterol? In addition to cholesterol, please watch out for the excess sodium found in meat dishes.[6] Extra sodium in your body leads to high blood pressure, which forces the heart to work harder and can lead to heart failure. Life is short, don't mess it up by eating meat. You need your heart; it is literally all that is standing between you and the Grim Reaper, so please "treat yourself" to a healthy lifestyle.

3. <u>Your Penis</u>. Many guys still buy the line "Real men eat meat." Even if you don't want to change your eating habits for your health, would you consider doing it to improve your sex life? Just like in the previous two points, the difference between healthy and unhealthy is all about blood circulation. Healthy blood flow means you are healthy enough to "get your freak on." Poor blood flow means you have ED (Erectile Dysfunction), a condition of not being able to "rise to the occasion."[7] Now you could pop some pills, but that is just a Band-Aid on the problem. Instead of a temporary solution, how about actually fixing the problem? Not only will you save money on medicine, but you will also get to have sex for many more years to come.

Eating Meat Negatively Affects:

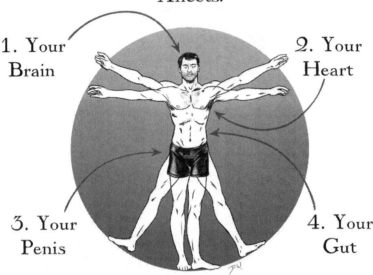

1. Your Brain

2. Your Heart

3. Your Penis

4. Your Gut

Going Vegan **CAN** help you avoid:

1. Obesity. There is a major link between the Standard American Diet and obesity. Excess pounds gained from an unhealthy diet exacerbate all medical ailments. Belly fat makes it difficult to walk, and if you walk with less frequency, you are more susceptible to weight gain. Extra weight adds pressure to your joints, which harms your back and knees. You should think of your heart like an engine, designed to move a train the size of your ideal body weight. When you gain weight, you increase the work load on your heart, without making the engine itself stronger. If you continue to increase the size of the train, you will eventually have a wreck on your hands. It doesn't have to be this way. Studies have shown "time and time again that vegetarians and vegans are slimmer than their meat-eating counterparts."[8] When it comes to your health, don't you want to be on the winning team?

2. <u>Cancer</u>. Eating meat has been linked to colorectal cancer. The American Cancer Society recently published an article about the World Heath Organization's finding of the correlation of animal eating and colon cancer. "Twenty-two experts from ten countries reviewed more than 800 studies to reach their conclusions. They found that eating 50 grams of processed meat every day increased the risk of <u>colorectal cancer </u>by 18%. That's the equivalent of about 4 strips of bacon or 1 hot dog. For red meat, there was evidence of increased risk of colorectal, <u>pancreatic</u>, and <u>prostate cancer</u>."[9] A plant-based vegan diet has been proven to be effective in cancer prevention. The Standard American Diet leads to colon cancer. The choice is yours. Which do you choose?

3. <u>Diabetes</u>. Per *The China Study*, "Both across and within populations, high fiber, whole, plant-based foods protect against diabetes, and high fat, high protein animal-based foods promote diabetes."[10] Diabetes is no joke. It's not the fact it kills you that scares me. SGT Vegan can live with death. What is scary about diabetes is that they have to cut little pieces of you off as your tissue dies. First you'll lose your toes, then your feet, then your legs. Diabetes is as sad as it is preventable. I have seen far too many patients suffering from the effects of untreated diabetes. It doesn't have to be this way. Studies have shown that a positive change in diet can not only reverse Type 2 (lifestyle related) diabetes, but also improve outcomes in cases of Type 1 as well.[11] (SGT VEGAN NOTE: Please check out the awesome book *Dr. Neal Barnard's Program for Reversing Diabetes*.)

You can dispute the results of findings from books such as *How Not to Die* and *The China Study*, but the facts are clear. Sure, your great-grandfather smoked two packs of cigarettes a day and ate cheesesteaks for breakfast all of his life and still lived to 100, but do you really think that is what is going to happen to you? Open your eyes and look around the next time you are at your favorite fast food stand or steak house. Does it look like the people around you will make it to 70, let alone 100? Now take a look at the yoga people who eat right. You are what you choose to eat. Break free from the Standard American Diet before it eats you alive, America!

ENVIRONMENT

It always surprises me when I talk to environmentalists who still eat meat. The facts are clear. "Animal agriculture is the leading cause of species extinction, ocean dead zones, water pollution, and habitat destruction."[12] It is hard to understand why environmentalists would support this industry by continuing to eat meat.

Champion of the environment, former Vice President Al Gore went vegan in 2013.[13] He explained the environmental argument for being vegan in an interview for *LateLine*: "It's absolutely correct that the growing meat intensity of diets around the world is one of the issues connected to this global crisis, not only because of the CO2 involved but also because of the water consumed in the process.."[14] Now that's an inconvenient truth!

Good work, Al. I'm glad you are more concerned with working to stop climate change than keeping rap music out of the hands of kids (SGT VEGAN NOTE: shameless 80's reference).

Here is the Environmental Argument for going vegan:

1. Animal Agriculture significantly contributes to global warming. At least 18 % of greenhouse gases are attributed to livestock.[15] Other estimates are as high as 51%, if you take into account the carbon footprint of everything needed to feed the cows and transport them to be killed for you to eat.[16] I turned to the Environmental Protection Agency for answers to the connection between Animal Agriculture and Climate Change. Before the current era of

governmental climate change denial beginning in January of 2017, the EPA had posted this factoid on its website to explain the negative effect of Animal Agriculture on the environment: "Livestock, especially cattle, produce methane (CH4) as part of their digestion. This process is called enteric fermentation, and it represents almost one third of the emissions from the Agriculture sector. The way in which manure from livestock is managed also contributes to CH4 and N2O emissions. Manure storage methods and the amount of exposure to oxygen and moisture can affect how these greenhouse gases are produced."[17] If you consider the mantra of supply and demand, the more we cut down on demand for animal flesh consumption, the more we cut down on the gases that are being created from the slaughterhouse death machinery.

2. Animal Agriculture is an inefficient use of water. "Meat and dairy production is more water intensive than crop production. For example, 500–4,000 liters of water are evaporated in producing one kilogram of wheat, depending on climate, agricultural practices, variety, length of the growing season and yield. However, to produce one kilogram of meat takes 5,000–20,000 liters, mainly to grow animal feed."[18] So in an American measurement system, they are saying one pound of meat, specifically cow flesh, takes between 600- 2401 gallons of water to make. That's about five times the amount needed for wheat. There are estimates that put the number as high as 12,007 gallons of water expended per pound of cow.[19] If those numbers seem unbelievable, consider what goes into them. When a calf is born it weighs between 60-100 lbs. After 18-22 months the average cows weigh between 1200-1400 lbs. To get to the point when they are ready to be "harvested" (SGT VEGAN NOTE: Animal Agriculture's term for slaughtered) cows have to eat loads of grain and drink a lot of water. You might be saying, "But what about my

protein?" Well, you could get all of your protein requirements from soybeans, (which only take 216 gallons of water to grow per pound), peanuts, legumes, or beans (Please see Part 2 for more information about Vegan Nutrition). The government subsidizes Animal Agriculture, which is why consumers don't pay the real cost of over $50 a pound for cow flesh at the supermarket. Clearly, raising cows just to be killed for food uses too many of our precious natural resources and is not sustainable for the environment and the planet.

3. We could stop world hunger overnight if we put an end to Animal Agriculture. "Some 40% of the world's land surface is used for the purposes of keeping all 7 billion of us fed...and the vast majority of that land — about 30% of the world's total ice-free surface — is used not to raise grains, fruits and vegetables that are directly fed to human beings, but to support the chickens, pigs and cattle that we eventually eat."[20] By ending the wasteful practice of raising animals for food, we would be able to grow enough grains to feed the entire population, SAVING the world for generations to come.

4. Animal Agriculture causes water pollution. In a 2000 report to Congress, the EPA determined about 40% of streams, 45% of lakes, and 50% of estuaries that were assessed were found to be polluted, and runoff from Animal Agriculture was a primary cause.[21] Animal excrement, urine, and all sorts of nasty chemicals come from farms and slaughterhouses and find their way into our lakes and streams. These vital waterways are being destroyed by Animal Agriculture, and instead of preventing this from happening our government continues to subsidize them. The more we continue to support that crappy industry (pun intended), the more polluted our water will become.

5. Animal Agriculture is responsible for the spread of disease. Mad Cow Disease (a direct result of raising cattle by feeding cow meat to cows) was a major factor in people 's

decision to stop eating cows during the outbreak several years ago. People often don't realize Animal Agriculture is responsible for spreading more diseases than just that one. "The World Organization for Animal Health estimates that no less than 60% of human pathogens and 75% of recent emerging diseases are zoonotic. Some human diseases have their known origins in animals, such as common influenza and small pox. Tuberculosis, brucellosis and many internal parasitic diseases, such as those caused by the tapeworm, threadworm, and so on, are transmitted through the consumption of animal products."[22]

Eating meat is poisoning the planet!

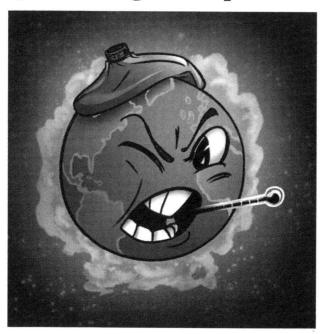

COMPASSION

"Compassion begins with the fork."

-Mohandas Gandhi

Sometime during human evolution, we domesticated animals. Some animals were chosen to be our companions, like the dog, while others were utilized for food, like the pig or the cow. Now we can spend our time playing video games and buying things we don't need rather than hunting and gathering food. While some would say this is progress, I argue that real progress would be for society to move beyond thinking of animals as a food source. Pigs, cows, chickens, dogs, and cats all have a right to exist beyond being raised for food.

Many "animal lovers" here in the West decry the eating of dogs in Asia while they themselves still eat other animals. They would make it illegal to hurt a dog, but still pay money to those who kill cows and pigs for them to eat. Pigs have the same intelligence as dogs, yet we pet one and kill the other. We excuse this inconsistency, stating it is "the way things are," but nothing could be further from the truth. The status quo remains this way because we allow it. In the 21st Century you can be anything you want to be, but you can't be an "animal lover" and still eat animals. That is illogical.

There are those who will inevitably counter by saying eating meat is "natural." Human teeth are not made to rip flesh from the bones of live prey like tigers, and our digestive tracks can't handle raw flesh the way carnivorous animals do. Modern society has manufactured cell phones, planes, and skyscrapers. We think and act the way we do because of conditioning, and that, in turn, becomes "natural" to us. If we can see the damage eating meat is causing our health, the planet, and other animals, we must choose to evolve beyond utilizing animals for food. That would be the "natural" choice.

The concept of "Humane Meat" is a myth people tell their children because they can't handle the brutality of the truth.

The packages of animal flesh organized in neat rows in your supermarket belies the torture and death they represent. Animals feel pain, and suffer immensely before they are killed. Slaughtering animals on behalf of those who refuse to give up eating animals is equivalent to a real-life horror movie. With all of the great vegan options these days, there is a better way for all of us to live.

There was a time when human beings had to eat meat to survive. Early man didn't have a steady source of food and was forced to eat meat. While we are no longer cavemen, many of us are still stuck in that old way of thinking. Eating meat has been ingrained into us from birth, and we are constantly bombarded with advertisements meant to keep us buying meat. However, we do have a choice. We can choose to continue to lie to ourselves about unhealthy eating habits which are destroying the planet and our bodies, or we can choose to face the facts. The choice is ours, and together we can make a change.

I ask you to choose compassion over killing. Choose a sustainable future for this planet. Choose a healthy lifestyle over one of obesity, cancer, and heart disease. Choose to evolve. Go Vegan.

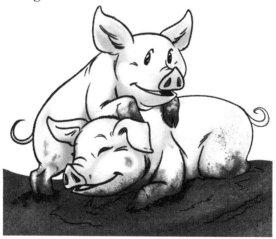

We Don't Need To Kill
What We Don't Need To Eat

Chapter 2

The Golden Age of Veganism

VEGANISM HAS COME A LONG WAY since I stopped eating meat in 1992. Back then, "vegan" was a dirty word, and the only people who identified themselves as vegans were punk rockers, hippies, and the Avant-garde. The early vegans had to be pioneers and create their own cuisine, because a lot of the things we now take for granted hadn't even been invented.

Veggie burgers did not yet exist. The closest thing we had was Nature Burger, and that was barely edible. You were better off with PBJs or just eating plain bread. Back then, plant-based milk was basically liquid tofu. We didn't have all of the varieties of milk substitutes we have now. My taste buds don't miss those days at all.

Suffice it to say, the vegan diet was limited in the early days, and most of us learned to cook out of necessity instead of a love for the culinary arts. We lived that way because we cared about animals and the environment. The vegan life wasn't easy in the pre-internet days and the negative public perception of vegans didn't win anyone over to a plant-based diet. We acted like martyrs and a lot of us looked like them, too. As a result, veganism went nowhere, the obesity epidemic only got worse, and climate change escalated. Luckily, most of that is in the past.

We've come a long way in a relatively short time. Being vegan doesn't mean being a culinary martyr anymore. I never thought I was going to be able to eat a cheese pizza again, and now there are several brands of vegan cheese (Daiya being arguably the most popular at time of writing). With vegan fast food joints and even vegan Dr. Martens shoes, anything you could ever want can be made vegan. There are even vegan options in Disneyland, which means vegans no longer have to go hungry in the happiest place on earth. Welcome to the Golden Age of Veganism.

All of the great, easily accessible products, coupled with the fact many celebrities are now vegan, has made being vegan into something of a trend. That is definitely okay by me. Any trend where the end goals are protecting animals, saving the planet, and eating healthier is the best thing ever. Being vegan is about making a better way to live on this planet, and everyone is welcome to join. We need to spread this message everywhere, not keep it to ourselves.

Unlike the other causes we have fought for in the last 50 years, veganism is a cause that makes looking good a priority. In a way, veganism sells itself if you do it right. If you look healthy, sexy, full of life and ready to kick ass, people will want to be more like you. At work, people are interested in hearing about what I eat not because they care about animals or the environment, but because I look good and they want to look good, too. If you look unhealthy, sickly or unhappy no one will want to come to Veganville, and the animals and planet will suffer as a result of it. Image is everything in the age of social media.

Veganism is not a cause that needs martyrs. We need less angst and more pictures of delicious plant-based foods spread all over the Internet. We need people talking about vegan athletes, and how you don't need to eat meat to build muscle and look great. We need more vegans that look good in bathing suits, more vegan movies stars and vegan celebrities. Yes, hurting animals and the planet sucks, but instead of making people feel bad, we need to make them feel GOOD about becoming vegan.

One thing the hippies did get right was positivity. Let's stay positive and work together to make the world a healthier, safer place for everyone, one delicious bite at a time. There has never been a better time to go vegan. If you are still on the fence about making the change, consider this: what do you have to lose but some inches off your waistline?

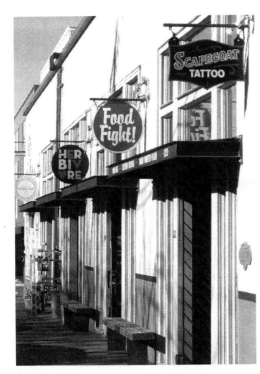

"Vegan Strip Mall, Portland, Oregon. Photo Courtesy of Stephanie Joy

Chapter 3

The Hidden Truth
of Animal Byproducts

IF YOU ARE NEW TO THE VEGAN GAME, you might be curious why vegans don't eat animal byproducts, such as eggs and milk. You might be saying to yourself, "Isn't it good enough to just be vegetarian?" Well, not to scare you off, but the answer is no.

Don't you think it's strange that humans are the only species who drink the milk from another completely different species of animal? Humans drinking cow milk makes as much sense as cows drinking our human mother's milk. Looking back in the full spectrum of stupid human history, from the institution of slavery to believing in witchcraft, just because people have been doing something for years does NOT make it right. Let me explain it in these terms: If eating meat supports the murder of animals, then drinking milk supports the RAPE and murder of animals.

The myth of Betsy the cow happily living life on the family farm is only a fairy tale people tell children because the truth is truly horrific.[23] Just like human beings, cows only naturally lactate (produce milk) around the time they have given birth for the purpose of nursing their babies. To keep up with high demands for milk production, cows in dairy farms are artificially inseminated on apparatuses called "rape racks."[24] The process involves shoving an arm up a cow's vagina to make sure the semen makes it to its destination inside the cow. When the cow has babies, those babies are sold as "veal." When cows are unable to give any more milk, they become "unhappy meals" themselves.

Drinking cow milk is healthy— if you are a baby cow. If you are a human, however, drinking milk is problematic for a variety of reasons. First, the hormones that are present in cow milk are meant to make a small calf become a huge cow. With the obesity epidemic a "big enough" problem already as it is in this country, I don't think we need people consuming something that will only exacerbate this problem even further.[25] In addition, cows are pumped full of antibiotics to keep them from getting sick at factory farms, and they pass that through their milk to humans, making some of the medical antibiotics we use in the hospital less effective. (SGT VEGAN NOTE: I don't want to go into a diatribe about the overuse of antibiotics, but you get the picture.) There is also a link between drinking cow milk and diabetes that deserves attention[26].

If you are drinking cow milk for the calcium, then you should know this: You don't need to! There are plenty of vegetable sources of calcium, such as fortified soy milk, beans, broccoli, and tofu, and if you are in doubt you can always take a vitamin supplement.[27] Hell, even OJ has calcium in it these days. Lastly, drinking milk has been shown to not effectively prevent osteoporosis.[28] Leave drinking milk for babies, who should drink their own mother's milk. (SGT VEGAN NOTE: Studies show babies drinking their mother's breast milk is good all around and vital to a baby's development --as long as the mother is not using drugs or HIV positive.)

Hens (female chickens) naturally produce eggs daily as a result of their menstrual cycle. If the hen mates with a rooster (male chicken), the eggs she produces during that time will be fertilized and eventually become baby chicks. If the hen doesn't mate with a male, she will just lay unfertilized eggs. These eggs are taken from the hens and eventually the hens themselves are killed and eaten when they can produce no more. To ensure the hens don't peck each other to death before they are killed, their beaks are clipped because living in slavery and waiting to die is stressful. The process couldn't be any more inhumane if Satan came up with it himself.

Medically speaking, the cholesterol found in all animal products is even more concentrated in egg yolks, because you are eating pure animal embryo. It might have a lot of protein in it, but it also is bad for you.[29] To summarize, both medically and ethically, when it comes to eating animal byproducts, "just say no."

Animal byproducts can be hidden in foods where you least expect them. You will always need to read the labels, but when you first go vegan, you are bound to make some mistakes. I wouldn't worry too much about it. Use all of the wonderful resources available to you (SGT VEGAN NOTE: Such as books like *Animal Ingredients A-Z*, and aps like *Is It Vegan?*) and try not to make the same mistake again. It will take a while before you are used to reading ingredients lists, and sometimes things will slip by. Cut yourself some slack. After all, we are only human, even when we are trying our best to be humane.

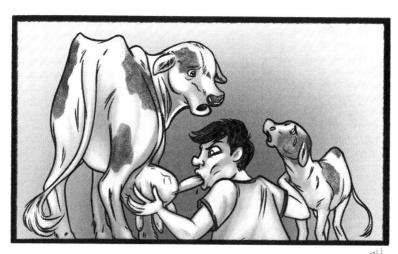

Drinking Milk is Weird

Chapter 4

Vegan Boot Camp

CONGRATULATIONS ON YOUR DECISION to go vegan! This is one of the most important choices you've ever made. In this chapter I break down "going vegan" into 3 easy-to-follow steps, along with 6 tips to make for a successful transition. While some people quit eating meat and go vegan "cold Tofurkey," I advise a well thought-out plan to ease your way into it.

You should transition from eating an animal-based diet to eating vegan at your own pace. The right way to go vegan is the way that is right for you. For myself, I started by cutting all red meat out of my diet, then seafood, then eggs, then cheese. From start to vegan took me about six months, but this could be done faster or slower depending on what is right for you. Work at your own pace and keep your eyes on the vegan prize.

Remember, you were raised eating meat and that is not your fault, nor is it the fault of your parents. Blame is unproductive and leads to resentment. None of us knew any better, and we need to forgive and forget. Now that you are moving towards living without the violence inherent in meat eating, you are making those steps toward a healthier, more compassionate lifestyle. The speed with which you take those steps is entirely up to you.

Becoming Vegan in Three Easy Steps:

Step 1: Stop eating meat. For some, this might be as easy as it sounds, and for others, this might be rather difficult. Begin by not eating cows and pigs. Once you are comfortable with not eating cows or pigs, proceed with not eating any meat at all. Work at eating more vegetables with every meal, and get excited about how you prepare them. Learn to substitute the meat in your dishes with plant-based proteins (see the cooking chapter for ideas), so you can still make the dishes you love without missing anything at all. Try to avoid eating extra dairy products or seafood in place of meat, as we will be working on eliminating those as well.

Step 2: Stop eating seafood. Some might call this stage the beginning of being vegetarian. Continue the good eating habits from Step 1, but begin to replace seafood with more plant-based foods, and eat more vegetables! If you are worried you are going to miss eating sushi, never fear! There are many delicious vegan items on the sushi menu. In fact, I usually gravitate towards going to sushi places when I go back to Japan as a visit, as a lot of the the dishes are made quick, cheap, delicious and vegan, and don't require making substitutions which might confuse a chef.

Step 3: Eliminate eggs and dairy from your diet. First, congratulations on becoming a vegetarian! This is an awesome accomplishment, and you should be proud of yourself for coming this far. Being vegetarian isn't difficult, but it does require dedication and intestinal fortitude to change, so be proud of yourself. Celebrate your transition to vegetarian, but don't get stuck there. A lot of people find giving up dairy products difficult, because they contain chemical compounds called "casomorphins," opiate-like molecules which makes them highly addictive.[30] I would start by getting out of the habit of eating dairy products by themselves. If you are a milk drinker, choose a plant-milk that works for you. I like soy the best, but if that's not your deal, you can also drink hemp milk, rice milk, coconut milk, almond milk, oat milk (big shout-out to Sweden's Oatly), or cashew milk. There are also many different cheese alternatives now, but they might take some getting used to. Most of these taste pretty good, but there will be a transition period during which your taste buds evolve. You have been used to eating and drinking things that come out of a cow's udder, after all, and since plants don't taste like cows they will taste somewhat different at first to you. After you have stopped eating dairy products as is, transition away from products that contain them, and begin baking and cooking with plant-based alternatives. Change is always a little hard, but cutting things out gradually will help you ease into the transition.

Congratulations on becoming Vegan! Keep up the great work! The rest of this book is written to support you. I've got your back.

Six Tips for the new Vegan:

1. You might feel hungry more frequently when initially transitioning to a vegan diet. That is normal. One reason for this is that it takes longer for your stomach to digest meat than it does plant matter. Another common cause of hungriness in people newly vegan is simply not eating enough calories. Remember, the diet part of "vegan diet" refers not to a unique way of starving yourself to lose weight, but a medical classification of a way to eat, such as a dialysis diet, cardiac diet, etc. I go into more depth about this later, but I generally recommend eating around 2000 calories a day, with as many calories as possible coming directly from plants, and limiting your intake of processed foods. If you are "feeling hungry all of the time," first make sure you are getting enough calories by adding up the

calories in all of the foods you are eating every day. If you aren't getting enough daily calories, simply eat more until you are eating AT LEAST_your minimum daily calorie requirement. Next, avoid foods that are highly processed or high in fat, salt, sugar - AKA junk food. Make sure you are drinking the recommended daily amount of water, two liters, which translates to 8 x 8oz glasses of water each day. You should be peeing clear. If your urine is yellow that could be a sign of dehydration. Water is not only necessary for your body to function properly, but it will also help with controlling hunger by filling up your stomach. Lastly, foods high in fiber will also help you feel full, so eat enough fiber without overdoing it, as it might give you the runs.

2. Get used to reading ingredients lists. I would literally spend hours reading ingredients lists when I first went vegan. Going grocery shopping with me was painful! I soon figured out what I could and couldn't eat. I also developed speed reading abilities in both Japanese and English. This is because your mind helps to point out key words, like animal names, milk, and other animal byproducts to make it easier to scan ingredients. Recently food shopping has gotten easier, with some products being labeled "vegan" by the Vegan Society (SGT VEGAN NOTE: You guys rule! Keep up the good work!). Also, common food allergens are now often listed on products in bold at the bottom of ingredient lists, so you can see which products have milk in them without your having to read the entire list. Lastly, there are apps you can get on your phone that will tell you if things are vegan or not with a barcode scanner. You should use them if they make your life easier, but for me, I'm just too old-school to need them.

3. Learn how to cook! It can be frustrating for your family to try to cook for you, so meet them halfway. Yes, everyone should be vegan, but don't be grumpy at your mom or

relatives just because they aren't ready to make vegan versions of your favorite meals for you. Volunteer to make great meals for your whole family to enjoy. The easiest thing to do when figuring out what to eat on a day-to-day basis is to veganize what you ate before you went vegan. For example, breakfast: oatmeal, or bagel, or cereal, pancakes, are mostly vegan or can be easily made vegan. Lunch: sandwich, drop the meat and cheese, add vegan substitute protein and you are good to go, or eat a salad without meat or cheese. As for dinner, the easiest would of course be pasta, which is often vegan by default, or rice/couscous (carbohydrate) with some sort of vegan protein and of course a gigantic portion of vegetables. Please see the cooking section for more ideas, and don't worry. Plenty of people go vegan everyday, and you can too!

4. <u>Try not to overdo it when you talk to about animal rights or the environmental impact of animal agriculture</u>. I understand the desire to tell everyone about *Earthlings, Cowspiracy, Forks Over Knives,* and every other documentary you just watched. I know that burning feeling to liberate every last tortured, enslaved, and abused animal because I feel it too. However, being a good vegan ambassador sometimes means getting along with meat-eaters just as much as it is about spreading the vegan message. Don't alienate people who are important in your life just because you have evolved and they haven't. I don't mean you should be wishy-washy or downplay your beliefs. A person should be able to stand firm and be able to respect others enough to agree to disagree. You are going to need to have patience and understanding when dealing with your friends and family. That will go a long way towards their acceptance of your beliefs. With widespread acceptance of veganism comes normalization, until finally compassion towards all lives becomes the new normal for everyone.

5. <u>Check with your family doctor if you have any specific medical questions</u>. Yes, being vegan can be the healthiest way to live, but no one is perfect and it never hurts to get a checkup every now and again. Getting yearly or bi-yearly blood work isn't a bad idea to make sure you aren't deficient in any nutrients. I also recommend a vegan multi-vitamin to everyone. The science is still out on their effectiveness (I talk more about this later), but it is a good, cheap insurance policy against possible deficiencies later, especially when it comes to Vitamin B-12.

6. <u>Don't throw out all of your non-vegan clothes overnight</u>. Not only is that not smart economically speaking, but it isn't great for the environment to add extra waste in a landfill either. Give them to friends or family members, sell them online, or replace them with compassionate alternatives as they wear out until you have an all-new vegan, earth friendly, kick-ass wardrobe!

Good luck in your transition to being vegan. I'll always be here for you if you have any questions.

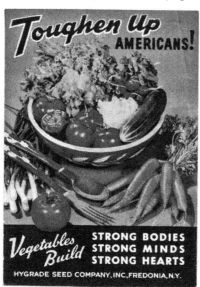

Courtesy of Miss Tia,
www.vintage-ads.livejournal.com

Chapter 5

Aquariums, Circuses, Zoos, and Hunting

AQUARIUMS, CIRCUSES, AND ZOOS are work camps for animals. I suppose these animals should be grateful they aren't being slaughtered outright like cows and chickens, but they are still prisoners suffering in captivity. If you want to see animals in their natural habitats, watch the *Nature Channel* or go on a hike somewhere away far away from human beings. Taking animals from their homes and putting them in cages just so people can conveniently gawk at them is inhumane. We've done a lot of horrible things in our relatively short existence as the human race, and now that we've technically put an end to human slavery (SGT VEGAN NOTE: let's not be naïve; it still exists in different forms) we should start working on ending animal slavery as well.

There have been some recent improvements in animal welfare. As a society we are becoming less tolerant of animal abuse. Stricter regulations for elephant trainers recently ended the reign of terror of a travelling circus company. The documentary *Blackfish* helped bring attention to the eco-treachery of a prominent aquatic theme park. Closing down these displays of human cruelty will go a long way in making a more caring and just world for all creatures. If you want to go to the circus, go to Cirque du Soleil. If you aren't a yuppie and still need to see some clowns, take a look at the Juggalos who follow the band Insane Clown Posse.

So what about hunting? Since the purpose of hunting is killing animals, should we consider hunting as bad as slaughterhouses? Considering their damage to the planet, slaughterhouses are worse for the environment than hunting. Also, given the nature of how the animals are killed, hunting animals in the wild is less cruel than killing them in slaughterhouses. Still, I don't think hunting should get a free pass on this one. There are better ways to live in the 21st century.

Modern day hunting, with its scoped rifles and camouflaged tree stands, shares more in common with snipers involved in military operations than it does with sports. In the military, we send snipers into battle to eliminate enemy targets while taking minimal risk to themselves. In war, you don't want your side to ever get into a "fair fight." You want overwhelming firepower and guaranteed wins leaving nothing to chance.

Sports, on the other hand, should be fair contests where the outcome is not decided before the match. In sporting contests there are winners and losers, and I don't think there are many human losers in this sport – unless you go hunting with Dick Cheney. Then you have about a 50-50 chance of being shot in the face.

If people want to keep calling hunting a sport, maybe we should arm the animals to make it fairer. Or hunters should go out like my father and use a flintlock rifle. He has only killed one deer with a flintlock rifle out of the twelve times he brought one hunting. It is some ancient technology and is so iffy that there is some actual skill to it. I can respect that, even if I don't agree with it.

Some hunters say shooting deer is the only way to keep the deer population under control. I would argue there are other more humane ways to limit the deer population, like sterilization and trap-and-release. We don't have to use killing as our default answer to every problem. There have been times in the past when we needed to use violence to right wrongs, such as in WW2, but there have been too many times in our recent history when we should have used our brains instead. Human beings need to learn to flex our heads as well as our muscles.

Zoos, Circuses, and Aquariums

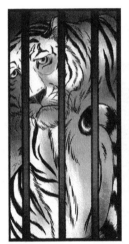 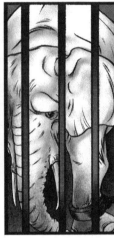 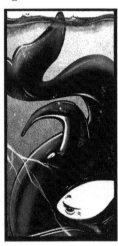

Chapter 6

Vegan Clothing

SINCE THE DAWN OF HUMANITY, people have been covering their genitals to protect against creepy crawlies and the elements. Almost immediately after Adam and Eve left the Garden of Eden, the first fashion designer started making clothes to meet this demand. At first, during the days of the hunter-gathers, people made clothes mostly out of the skins of the animals they had killed. As time went on, humans evolved into using cloth made from spun cotton. Cotton has been used for making clothing for about 5000 years, in ancient India, China, Egypt, and also Peru and Mexico. Of course, the cotton produced in the American South during the pre-Civil War days was horrible because it relied heavily on slave labor, and that issue was eventually sorted out with some war and a whole lot of death. These days, however, cotton is cruelty-free; since the production has become mechanized, neither human nor animal has to be hurt in its production. Demand for non-animal clothes has produced a number of inventions for clothes and footwear. This is a great time in human attire if you aren't into wearing animals.

Full disclosure: SGT Vegan isn't even remotely fashionable, unless you consider 80's New York Hardcore fashionable, in which case, I'm straight up couture. My fashion evolution ended long ago with cut-off camouflage shorts, a punk rock t-shirt and running shoes. I wear scrubs to work, don't shave, and while I was in the Army, I literally wore the same thing every day. In other words, unless you are preparing for battle either in Afghanistan or in a Cro-Mags mosh pit, I have no advice to give you on fashion. Taking fashion advice from me would be like having Jabba the Hutt as your personal trainer. (SGT VEGAN NOTE: Please excuse the *Star Wars* reference). I can point you in the right direction towards some cool vegan clothing companies, and some on-line vegan stores you may not have heard of, so let's get started!

Here is a list of some vegan clothing stores and outfitters, and vegan clothing designers that you might find helpful. I borrowed this list from the Farm Sanctuary website; please check them out at www.farmsanctuary.org and donate!

Vegan designers and brands:

- ▶ Vaute (vautecouture.com). NYC based vegan boutique clothing store. Mostly for women – jackets, dresses, shirts, jewelry and accessories.
- ▶ Love is Mighty (loveismighty.com) – Women's shoes.
- ▶ Brave Gentle Man (bravegentleman.com). High-end NYC based men's clothing store. I like how they add "future" to traditional animal-based products to mean vegan versions of something, like "future leather," or "future wool." Just when you think you know it all, someone comes up with something new and cool.
- ▶ Matt & Nat (mattandnat.com) – High-end bags and pocketbooks for women.
- ▶ Susan Nichole (susannichole.com) - Wallets and handbags for women.
- ▶ Gunas (gunasthebrand.com) - Women's handbags
- ▶ OlsenHaus (olsenhaus.com) - Women's' shoes and more.
- ▶ NOHARM (noharm.com) - High end Italian men's and women's shoes and accessories.

- Vegetarian Shoes (vegetarian-shoes.co.uk) - Men's and women's shoes and accessories. I've worn the boots before and they are comfortable and well-made. I still have a vegan "future leather" jacket back from my punk rock era. Understand that the prices are in English pounds, so they might be expensive, depending on the exchange rate.
- You can also get vegan Dr. Martens boots now. The 4 - eye shoes fit my feet weird, but the 8- eye boots are comfortable right out of the box. Look on Dr. Marten's website, but you can buy them cheaper on Amazon.

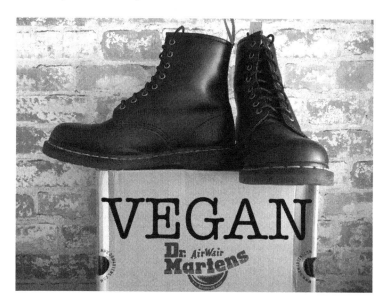

One- stop vegan shop:

- Mooshoes NYC/LA (mooshoes.com) - They carry many vegan brands for shoes and shirts, and have cool in-store events. I've been to both stores, and really like what they do.
- Vegan Essentials (veganessentials.com) - Complete vegan online store, with products from clothes to food. If it's vegan, you can buy it here.

▶ Vegan Chic (veganchic.com) - Vegan Fashion online store.
▶ Alternative Outfitters (alternativeoutfitters.com)- CA-based vegan fashion boutique.
▶ Herbivore Clothing (herbivoreclothing.com) – A Portland-based store full of t-shirts, hoodies, stickers and accessories.

Cheaper Alternatives:

▶ Payless Shoes. Has a lot of cheap, non-leather shoes. Not always the best quality, but at least they are affordable, and animal-free.
▶ Army-Navy Surplus Stores. Some of the military dress shoes with the "permanent- shine" are vinyl and not leather. Check out your local military or law enforcement supply store to buy them.

In conclusion, wear what you want, but when you buy new clothes, please buy animal and sweatshop-free clothing. None of this has to break the bank, and there are plenty of great cruelty-free products out there everywhere.

Chapter 7

Vegan in the Army

(SGT Vegan WARNING:
Contains Army language. Reader discretion advised!)

I GRADUATED FROM THE University of Pittsburgh with a dual degree in Japanese and Sociology. What do you do for a job after majoring in such a random collection of subjects? I didn't know either, so I moved to Japan to find out. For someone who speaks the language and has a sense of adventure, Japan is an awesome place to live. I loved getting out of my comfort zone, meeting people from all over the world, and making easy money teaching English. Tokyo was a great place to get gigs on TV shows, to see bands play, and eventually form a band of my own. Being in a band was a lot of fun, and eventually led to me performing on the *Final Fantasy X* videogame soundtrack (a story for another day). I had a second, and maybe third childhood in Japan, continuing my carefree years of college. Y2K was supposed to end the world, but for me the good times kept rolling on. Life couldn't get any better.

9/11 changed everything. I was walking home from work that night when I got an emergency text from the Japanese government saying there was a big fire in a New York building. I was wondering what that meant, when I got a call from a friend who explained the World Trade Center had been attacked. I spent the rest of the night at my neighbor's apartment, glued to the TV screen, in absolute horror of what was happening to our world. The good times were officially over.

The day before I was loving my life as an ex-pat in Japan, zero responsibilities and carefree, and now I was feeling guilty for it. Much like when the Greatest Generation answered the call after Pearl Harbor, I also felt compelled to do something. I started by putting on benefit shows for the children of the victims of the 9/11 attacks. As time progressed America started bombing the hell out of Afghanistan, so I divided the money I raised between the children of the victims of 9/11 victims and Afghan children who were orphaned due to the war. I felt like that was better than nothing, but it still wasn't enough. As crazy as it might sound, I felt like I personally had been called to do more, so I left my easy life in Japan to figure out what that was.

At first I tried to join the FBI, but I was disqualified because I had been living outside of America for too long. My next choice was the military. I had thought about going into the military before, but I had given up on the idea when I went vegan. My big hang-up with the military was having to wear leather combat boots, but since the world was coming to an end that didn't seem to matter as much anymore. I decided I would help make the world a better place by serving my country in the Army. I couldn't stop the world from being at war, but I would be able to save lives on both sides by serving as a medic. I vowed whatever happened, I would remain true to my values and serve my country with honor.

I went through basic training (also known as boot camp) in January 2003 at Ft. Benning, GA. Boot camp sucks for everyone, but it is especially hard on vegans. Vegan options? Minimum. I had to fight with the assholes running the chow hall (cafeteria) every day just to get an extra scoop of peanut butter. I ate salad sandwiches, calling them "BLTs"" (bread, lettuce, tomato). I breakfasted with Tony the Tiger, eating my

Frosted Flakes in orange juice because soymilk wasn't available. Did I get enough calories? Fuck no I didn't! I ate just enough to keep me alive, but I felt like shit, working out 16 hours a day on less than 1500 shitty calories. Things got a little better toward the end, because we mostly ate Meals Ready to Eat (MRE's). MRE's guaranteed peanut butter packs a plenty, mixed fruit, and even a bean burrito that was accidentally vegan (later to be replaced by the shitty, non-vegan veggie burger).

I soon came to realize that if not for the food aspect, boot camp would have been pretty awesome. Boot camp is kind of like an all-included resort vacation. All of your activities are planned for you, it includes free meals and lodging, and all you have to do is show up. You essentially get paid to hang out, work out and shoot guns. What's not to love about that?

Unfortunately, every meal in boot camp is a struggle if you are vegan, and always being hungry made those stressful times even harder. Still, I got through it, you can too if you decide to go down that rabbit hole. I'm guessing being vegan would be even easier in the Navy and probably super easy in the Air Force. In the "Chair Force" you just ask your waiter for the vegan options on the menu!!! (SGT VEGAN NOTE: Just kidding, but not really, the Air Force is notoriously cushier than the other branches.) In the Marines, being vegan might even be harder than in the Army, but who knows? Neither branch is known as a bastion of free-thinkers.

After boot camp comes AIT, Advanced Individual Training. For me, that meant going to Ft. Sam Houston to become a medic. I loved being a medic. As a "save the world" type of person, it was a job that gave me a mission in line with my personal views of the world. I was going to be able to help everyone, both the people we might be fighting, and the soldiers I was serving with. I suffered from the effects of malnutrition for weeks after boot camp ended, but I eventually got better. Ft. Sam was a training camp for both sexes, and even had veggie burgers in the cafeteria! And, unlike boot camp, we were free to go off base during non-training hours. I went to Austin whenever I could, ate vegan Chinese food, and shopped at the local commissary (SGT VEGAN NOTE: Army talk for supermarket). In a month, I was back to my normal self. I was in great shape, getting through the grueling pace of learning the medic stuff, and eating like a champ. Thanks US ARMY!

While at Ft. Sam Houston I volunteered to be a Ranger, an action which I blame on the movie *Black Hawk Down*. The Rangers are badass, a tier of the "Special Operations" community, and of course, I wanted in. Even the act of volunteering to be a Ranger is a little dramatic. You have to go to a special office on base where they look through your personnel file to make sure you are eligible. Then you have to sign a waiver. No rights for you anymore; a complete blank check written to the US Government. I meditated on a recruitment poster I saw on the wall advertising the Rangers. It featured an intimidating soldier with an M16 and a quote mistakenly attributed to George Orwell. I pondered the words "People sleep peaceably in their beds at night only because rough men stand ready to do violence on their behalf," while the clerk in charge ripped up my original contract and told me I would be heading to the Ranger Indoctrination Program after Airborne School.

I was apprehensive to return to Ft. Benning for Airborne School. It had taken me months to get over the damage the "Boot Camp Diet" had caused me, and I was not excited to go back to starving every day. Lucky for me, Airborne School turned out to be more like the resort vacation I had dreamed about. No responsibilities, 9-5 training, and we were able to come and go as we pleased as long as we made it to formation on time. (SGT VEGAN NOTE: Formation is Army-talk for troops formally lined up and in uniform. Failure to make any formation times would result in me being kicked out of Airborne School.) Other than the risk of injury that came from jumping out of planes, life was pretty easy. I had the extra energy to go back to working out in my free time, and I was eating like a fucking champ.

In the beginning, I was happy just to have access to a steady supply of vegan food, but of course I soon had to push the boundaries of my new freedom to the limits. I came up with a cunning plan – I would fly back home to Philadelphia, retrieve my car, and drive it back to base. With a car, the whole world would be open to me and there would be nowhere I couldn't go and nothing I couldn't do. The idea was solid, and the plan – a one-way ticket to Philly and a long drive back to base – was simple enough.

The plan almost took a detour towards oblivion when I agreed to drop my father and sister off along the way so they could do some hiking. One of my family's quirks is a love that borders on obsession with outdoor adventure. When my Dad heard I would be driving back to Georgia, he immediately enlisted me to help him in his eternal quest to check more miles off of the Appalachian Trail. The Appalachian Trail, also known as the AT, is a 2,200 mile hiking trail that stretches from Maine all the way to Georgia. My dad had been slowly hiking the AT in sections for the better part of a decade. Since I was driving south towards Georgia anyway, I would only have to go "a few short miles" out of my way to be able to help them out.

I was apprehensive because I had to drive about 800 miles to get back to base, and I had a formation at 05:00 in the morning. While the task bordered on the impossible, I'm an optimist and "a few short miles" didn't sound too bad. Looking at my dad's map, I reasoned I would only be going about an inch out of my way. What could possibly go wrong?

Of course, few plans ever go the way you expect them to. The drive started out easy enough. We were taking the highway back and we had left with plenty of time to spare. The problem arose when we realized the inch out of my way was not made up of highways, but of winding mountain roads with very low speed limits. Suddenly, my time advantage vanished and I was up against a time crunch. When I dropped them off so they could start their hike, I realized I was now 5 hours out of my way. I barely had a snowball's chance in hell to make it back on time, let alone early. I drove straight through the night, only stopping for gas along the way. I pulled into Ft. Benning at 04:55, changed into my uniform in the parking lot, and made it to formation just as my name was called. I ran the 5 miles that followed roll call with my eyes closed and a smile on my lips, happy to not be kicked out of Airborne School.

After Airborne School, I spent two months in Airborne Hold. Airborne Hold means you are still a part of the Airborne School unit, but since you aren't training you are forced to spend your days doing chores for the Army (called details). One such detail we had was to work at the CQ (charge of quarters) desk for 24 hours and do random bullshit, like answer phones, or be a "Gofer" (As in "go for this fucker, go for that shithead"). The good part of this duty was after working for 24 hours straight, a soldier was then free to do whatever they wanted for the next 2 days. I usually spent my free time hanging out in the Atlanta or eating at Country Life, a 7th Day Adventist vegetarian cafe. I enjoyed their delicious vegan food and loved chatting with all of the hippies and seniors who spent their days there. I also hung out with my buddy Zach, who had gone AWOL after his first week of Airborne Hold.

One day after doing 24-hour CQ duty, I overheard someone in charge bark that anyone going to the Ranger Indoctrination Program (RIP) was to report immediately to the hospital to get their Ranger Physical. Not wanting to get caught in this web of Army fuckery and lose the free time I had just earned, I immediately got in my car and raced off base so I could deny hearing the order. After all, original intelligence said we would be leaving sometime in the next couple of weeks, so I could get this physical anytime. I had a great weekend on the town, and crashed at Zach's place. You might call this sort of behavior "irresponsible," but after being treated like the

Army's bitch you start to fight back any way you can to keep your sanity and a little bit of dignity.

When it was time to return, I made sure I stopped at the hospital and got my Ranger Physical. Of course, I was in great shape, so the physical was just a formality for me. When I was done I drove back to the barracks. I was sleepy because we had been up all night driving around and getting into trouble. I was hoping for a super-chill day so I could take a nap and get my stuff ready for RIP.

Let me explain what I meant by "getting my stuff ready." When one goes to a training scenario in the Army, there is always a contraband shakedown. The official reason for the shakedown is for safety. Instructors look for guns, knives, nunchucks, drugs and anything else that you could hurt yourself or others with. While that's the official reason, it is really just an opportunity to fuck with people. Drill Sergeant types inspect your gear and confiscate anything out of the ordinary. (SGT VEGAN NOTE: I once had my vegan Bacon Bits confiscated during a health and welfare inspection in Medic Training. "Muir! What the fuck is this?! "Bacon Bits, Drill Sergeant!! They make my salads more fun!!") I was determined not to allow that to happen again. I was going to go through my locker and take out anything which might get the attention of the cadre, then hide it in my car. This was going to be the easiest shakedown ever! Best thing of all, I had at least three days to get this done. I was going to make sure I had the most army-regulation locker ever!

I pulled up into the barracks parking lot and turned off my car. I was about to get out of when I noticed some guys from my unit were in formation. I sat for a minute trying to figure out what they might be doing there, and what I should do. It was too early for them to be going off to work, and some of those guys out there should have also been exempt after having just gotten off 24-hour details. Then I realized that this was the group being readied to go for Ranger Training. They were leaving early!! I was supposed to be there with them, but I was not ready. I was sitting in my car doing the wrong thing. This was not good. I was fucked. "Fuckfuckfuckfuckfuckfuckfuck" I muttered to myself, hoping in vain this yogic-like chanting would make the problem go away. I sat there debating my options. Quickly, I decided I should do the noble thing and escape. I turned the car back on, trying to be as quiet as possible, as if my car would know we were now in stealth mode. I was putting the car in reverse when I locked eyes with one of the instructors (also called cadre). He thundered my name. "Muirrrrrrrrrrr!!!!" I could hear him though the closed car windows. There was no getting around it. I was screwed.

Dejectedly, I got out of the car and approached the formation. A bunch of my friends were lined up with a very unfriendly looking man standing in front of them.

"Muir! Where the fuck were you?"

"Getting my physical, Sergeant."

"You were supposed to get that shit already, fuck face!"

"I had 24 hour CQ before that, and I had the day off."

" Bullshit! You should have known that you had to get your physical before today. "

"I didn't know, SGT!" (SGT VEGAN NOTE: This was a lie.)

"OK! Grab your shit out of your locker, and get the fuck in formation." He gestured at a couple of my comrades. "Go help him."

While my flimsy excuse for not already having my physical had somehow worked, the worst was yet to come. Getting my things together was a cluster fuck at best. My locker contained a mishmash of food, porn, appliances (a blender for making post workout protein shakes), video camera, pictures, letters from my family and girlfriend, candy, assorted coins, vegan Bacon Bits, and knives. There was stuff everywhere, and it took two of my friends to help me to with the bags. Eventually I made it to formation and I walked with everyone all of the way to the Ranger compound, which turned out to be next door.

We stood spread out in a sandbag-walled area of blacktop about the size of a basketball court. The Ranger flag, with the

75th training emblem on it, flew ominously over head. A Ranger instructor walked in front, glaring at us.

"Alright fuck faces. You have two minutes to take everything out of every bag. Two fucking minutes. Make it happen. Go!"

I opened my bags. I had a thousand things in bags, most of them in multiple bags. I worked as fast as I could, but time ran out and we were doing push-ups again.

We continued to play this game, until finally I was the only one who still hadn't taken everything out of the bags. All attention turned towards me, and two of the cadre moved over my way to "help" me with my bags. By "help" I mean they threw all of my stuff everywhere, while they "helped" themselves to my food, looked through my photos, and yelled in my face every step of the way. I was in awesome shape so the exercise didn't phase me, and sooner or later I got all of my shit squared away (SGT VEGAN NOTE: Army talk for "completing a task."). An hour later, in the middle of the smoke session (SGT VEGAN NOTE: Army talk for performing calisthenics for an unknown length of time, usually to complete exhaustion.) one of the guys started to cry, and I smiled, for I knew I was no longer at the top of the shit list.

I thought I was completely out of the Cadre's shitlight, when one of the cadre noticed the vegan tattoo on the back of my neck. "Mother-fucker! This asshole's a vegan!" The cadre discussed what a vegan was, and my imminent demise was decided upon. A flurry of pushups, sit-ups, and more creative exercises ensued.

When enough time had elapsed, we were brought into a classroom and filled out paperwork. We also had a few speeches by the Ranger training staff, and the commander of the battalion. The commander began his speech, " Men! Rangers are not fucking soldiers. Rangers are fucking killers." He had everyone stand up, and ask him a question one by one. My question, of course, was if vegans were allowed to be Rangers. "How the fuck should I know? They have vegetarian

MREs, so why the fuck not?" That was good enough for me. I vowed to make it through this course. We headed back to the blacktop, and the Ranger cadre was pissed. I was fired up, though, and could take it. With that out of the way, the rest of the day was easy.

In the following weeks I was harassed every day for being vegan. I didn't care. I took all of their verbal abuse in stride, for I had skin thicker than a rhino's. RIP itself wasn't too bad. We spent all day working out, but I would have been doing that as a civilian anyway. Our uniform called for us to wear a two-quart canteen, which I quickly drained of water and started to use as a secret hiding place for my vegan cream cheese so my bagels wouldn't have to be lonely during breakfast. The chow hall here did not have veggie burgers, but it had a great salad bar, and an unlimited amount of peanut butter. I wasn't losing any weight, at least. Then on our jump day (out of a plane) I admitted to using my cell phone to call my girlfriend and I was immediately kicked out of the program. I was pretty angry with the Army, to be cut from the program for something so trivial. I couldn't help but think they were using this minor infraction as an excuse to get rid of the vegan, since they couldn't eliminate me based on my performance.

I spent the next couple of months hanging out with the other RIP failures. We had volunteered to become Rangers, and despite giving 120% effort that hadn't happened. We had, instead, become the Army's servants in RIP Hold. Other than the fact we were in America and it wasn't WW2, RIP Hold felt like a real-life version of the war sitcom *Hogan's Heroes*. We turned our attention to the job of avoiding bullshit, which we vowed to excel at. We were friends with the squad leader, and made sure he gave our tight knit group the job of cleaning the gym. We found a hidden room where we could avoid the leaders and assorted bullshit. We only left our clubhouse when it was time to work out or occasionally clean gym equipment. We played cards, read magazines, and hung out like the kids in *Stand By Me*.

This chapter of my Army experience was a waste of time. I hadn't joined the Army to sit around or hang out; I had joined the Army to save the world. I started to get antsy and demoralized. Months went by. I reapplied for RIP and was turned down. It became easier to get vegan food, but I didn't join the Army for the food, and I didn't want to just survive, I wanted to thrive! Then, one day, all of the waiting ended.

I was in the hideout busy doing nothing when a runner barged through the door. I glared at him.

"What do you want, fucker?"

"They are calling for you in formation. Looks like they have orders for you and a couple others."

"Fuck off."

"No. For real."

I went to investigate. Sure as shit, the staff sergeant in charge of RIP holdovers was holding orders. He saw me.

"Muir, get the fuck up here."

I ran up and got my assignment.

"173rd Airborne. Vicenza, Italy." I was going to Italy. Fuck yes!

The first thing I did when I got to Italy was to figure out how I could move off-post so I had my own kitchen. Normally people at their first duty stations don't get to live off-post, but I had an "in." I joined forces with a guy I knew from Airborne School who was allowed to move off-post on the condition he could find a roommate. We couldn't have been more different. He was a by- the- books neat freak, and I was a messy vegan punk rocker. Still, neither of us wanted to be living on- post, so I had a doctor to write me a note stating I needed to have access to a kitchen in order to stay healthy. I learned from experience I was going to have to set myself up for success by any means necessary, and suffering in silence was not going to get this mission accomplished.

I started to go out on the town and get some good vegan food. Italy is very vegan friendly. Vegan pizza? Check. Cheap and delicious pasta? Of course. Vegan soy gelato? Yes, oh fuck yes, by the kilo- 2.2 lbs. a week, baby! In boot camp I had lost a lot of weight, and I now had the opposite problem. A pizza a day is arguably too much food, and the hazelnut soy ice cream I was chasing it down with wasn't helping to keep the weight off. Luckily, I was running an average of 5 miles a day and lifting weights. After a couple of weeks in Rear Detachment my unit returned from Iraq. As you would guess from any military movies you might have seen, the new guys get fucked with, especially the vegan ones. This is the unstated law of the land. Still, I was an ok medic and in really good shape. My PT score spoke for itself. I've always taken being in shape seriously, and since now I was moving towards combat I doubled my efforts, working out with my unit and on my own.

After a fun year in Italy eating, sightseeing and training, I deployed to Afghanistan in March of 2005. My year in Afghanistan will always be a part of me, even though the experience now seems surreal and more like something out of a movie than my actual life. I think my mind sometimes dwells on that time due to the survivor's guilt of making it while others didn't. There wasn't any rhyme or reason. Things just happened, and fair didn't have anything to do with it.

As to how I stayed vegan in a warzone, I started off by sending myself a bunch of food before I even left. I was attached to an artillery unit, and would not be moving around as much as I would have if I were with an infantry unit, which meant I could hoard food if I could get my vegan hands on some. On my first day in country my Platoon Sergeant informed me one of the boxes I had sent myself here had exploded in transit. Apparently I looked at him in disbelief as I said back to him "Exploded?!" while making a hand gesture of an explosion, which was the source of jokes given all of the deadly "explosions" in Afghanistan.

I didn't know what I was going to do once I ran out of food. We had a chow hall, but other than bagels and salad I was shit out of luck. Once I realized a lot of the food the locals were eating was vegan by default I worked out a barter system to stay fed. I traded locals for halal meals (MREs for Muslims), and ate at the chow hall for locals, but I soon got in trouble for doing that and had to find another way.

Luckily someone told me about anysoldier.com, a website for deployed service members. I put a post up about some things my guys needed, and mentioned I was vegan. The floodgates opened and the vegan food came pouring in. I ate like a king for the rest of my deployment as a result. Through the intervention of my friend Dana I also came to be supported by Tofurkey. They sent me many boxes of their shelf stable, vegan products, and I sent them some pictures of myself with holding the Tofurkey with a 105 mm howitzer and a mountain in the background. That picture went on their website and was one of the top images of "Vegan Power" on Google search at the time.

Toward the end of my deployment I had to tell people not to send me any more food. I ate my stash down to the point where the only thing left was cans of chili. I had chili stacked from the floor to the ceiling in the hooch (our makeshift living quarters, made out of plywood). Every day I would wake up and grab another can. Sooner or later I just stopped wanting to eat. Till this day, I still avoid chili if I can help it.

So did I maintain my vegan status while in Afghanistan? Yes, with the exception of one situation that was beyond my control. One day I got word we were heading out of the wire on a mission, and we had to be prepared to be out for a couple of days. I had gone on missions before, but they were usually short, and I didn't worry about anything besides my gear. In this case, I had to pack up food, bandages, bullets, uniforms, and we had a 20-minute timeline to work with. Halfway through packing, one of the soldiers hit his head on the howitzer, and it left a big gash that required stitches. I stopped what I was doing and stitched up his head, and then went back to preparing for the mission. By the time I was done I had enough vegan food, med supplies, and bullets socked away for a couple of days.

Little did I know, this was Operation Red Wings. If you've seen the movie or read the book *Lone Survivor*, you know there was a lot going on. My platoon's particular piece of this puzzle was to provide fire support for the ongoing rescue operation of a Navy SEAL. As a medic I was lucky, because my main job was to take care of the guys who got sick while we sat in a field for weeks with temperatures as high as 130 degrees Fahrenheit. As a vegan, though, I wasn't so lucky. As days turned to weeks, my Cliff bars quickly ran out, and I had to rely on a dwindling supply of MREs.

MREs were fun at first, and had endless mixing combos. Trading with the guys reminded me of hustling baseball cards as a kid. Unfortunately, there were only a very limited amount of the bean burrito MREs. When that ran out, I rat fucked (SGT VEGAN NOTE: this means to search all of the containers, opening up every package until you get what you want) all of the wheat snack bread, peanut butter and fruit cups I could get my hands on. Later, towards the end of the mission, shooting all day and sleeping in foxholes at night (SGT VEGAN NOTE: foxholes are small holes about the size of a shallow grave we dug in the ground to protect ourselves from enemy fire, should there be any), the vegan options ran out completely.

Realizing I could not live for very long on Charms (the hard candy in the MREs, fuck you Charms!), I had to suck it up and eat the pasta with vegetables MRE, a vegetarian meal which contained a small amount (less than 2% if you can believe the package) of egg whites. The choice I had before me was to either get enough calories to fuel my brain so I could do my job while slightly compromising my principles, or to put lives at risk by starving until the mission was over. I chose to eat the pasta, and we all lived to tell the tale. Therein lies the lesson of being vegan: You do the best you can in every situation, and always keep moving forward.

DEPARTMENT OF THE ARMY
HEADQUARTERS AND HEADQUARTERS COMPANY
1ST BATTALION (AIRBORNE), 508TH INFANTRY
Vicenza, Italy
APO AE 09630

1 FEB 2005

AESE-PCC-H

SUBJECT: MEMORANDUM FOR RECORD

1. The following soldier, SPC William Muir ▓▓▓▓▓▓▓ will be placed on a Vegan Diet.

2. Vegan Diet: SPC Muir cannot consume animal or animal product foods. (i.e. eggs, fish, poultry, meat, and diary products)

3. POC for this memorandum is the undersigned at 634-6633.

Edward A. White, D.O.
MAJ, MC
Battalion Surgeon

Edward A. White, D.O.
FEB – 1 2005
MAJ US Army MC

SGT Vegan's Dr. Note.

47

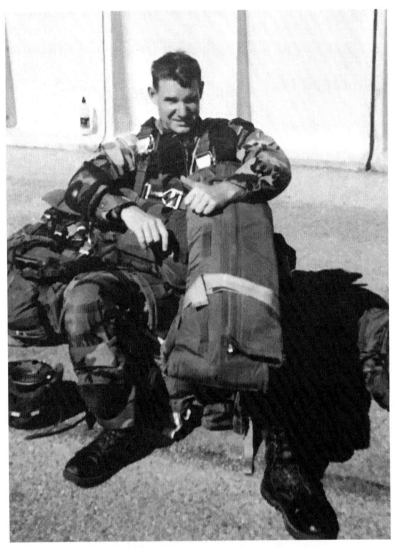

**SGT Vegan waiting to jump into action
with the 173rd Airborne Brigade**

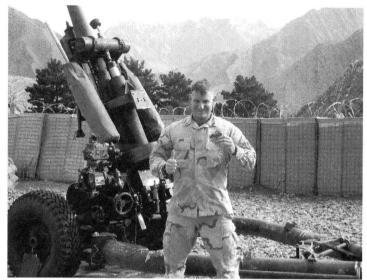

Tofurkey and Howitzers

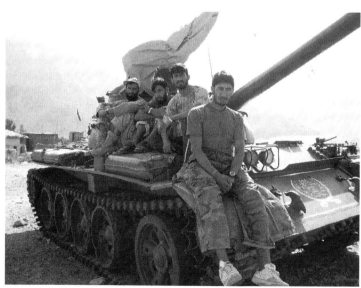

Afghan National Army, 2005

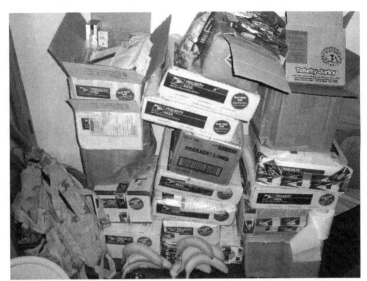

Thank you anysoldier.com and anyone who sent me food in while I was in Afghanistan.

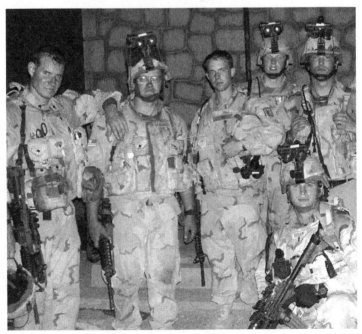

Delta Battery, 1st Platoon

Chapter 8

Vegan During the Holidays

HOLIDAYS AND SPECIAL OCCASIONS are stressful times for everyone, but they can be even worse if you have to figure out what you are going to eat while dealing with non- supportive friends and family members. Many non-vegans, especially the over 50-year-old members of your family, might not be able to comprehend the break in tradition which comes with not eating something because it includes animals. Or they might say: "The stuffing isn't made with meat," they will say, "just chicken." "The bread doesn't have animals in it- just eggs and milk; that's ok, right?" Think back to the way you used to think to get where they are coming from.

A Vegan Zombie Returns Home For The Holidays

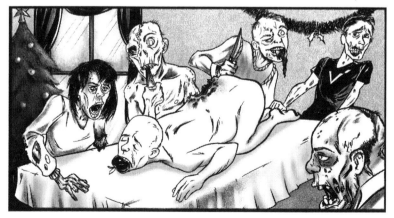

At least 99% of us ate meat growing up, so it shouldn't be hard to remember. A little bit of patience and planning ahead goes a long way towards a Happy Holidays for all.

5 Vegan Tips for Surviving the Holidays

1. Bring your own food. A sure fire way to guarantee something gets done right is to do it yourself. Thanks to Tofurkey, and a hundred other companies just like it, you can easily bring your main course with you. You can probably even heat it up where you are going to be eating with carnivorous relatives: just remember to bring your own dish and have aluminum foil on hand to keep food separated.

2. Check and see if any of the side dishes can be made vegan long before the day of the event. There is no good reason you can't substitute Earth Balance (a delicious, buttery plant-based vegan margarine) for butter in a recipe for vegetables that is otherwise vegan if you supply the Earth Balance yourself. Don't get ahead of yourself and think your relatives are going to do that for everything, though. Be realistic, and limit your requests, and there is a better chance there will be compliance with your vegan wishes.

3. Ask to bring a desert for everyone to share. Vegan Apple Pie vs. Animal Apple Pie? Who can tell the difference? Nobody can! Bring your own ice cream to put on it, and don't expect anyone to choose soy/coconut ice cream over cowtit milk...because cowtit milk isn't gross like the other one. Sarcasm, of course!

4. Stick to your guns, but be nice about it. Nobody cares you are vegan, even if it is better for the animals, health, and the planet...especially during the Holidays. People just want to stuff their faces and open presents. So don't bother bringing it up, and be nice. That being said, don't play the "when in Rome" crap and eat turkey/ham/a cat because you are at your Grandma's and don't want to stand up for yourself. Grow a spine! People often see others being

vegan as a questioning of their own values. You don't have to be self-righteous about other people's refusal to change, but you DO need to stand firm and be true to your own values. Cave to peer pressure and people will hold that over your head for the rest of your life.

5. Remember to have fun and enjoy the holidays. Set yourself up for success so being vegan looks easy. Have great food, and be happy eating it, and people will be interested in what you are doing and consider the merits. If you make being vegan into a "martyr act," you limit the opportunities of being a good vegan ambassador when it really counts. Being grumpy isn't very attractive, and it isn't much fun, either.

Chapter 9

Vegan Road Trip

I DO A TRAVEL FOOD VIDEO BLOG called Vegan Road Trip. I travel all over the world, and find delicious vegan food most everywhere I go. Preparation and know-how can go a long way towards success when it comes to going on a Vegan Road Trip. Let me share with you some tricks to having a successful one.

1. Choose your destination wisely. Some destinations are more vegan-friendly than others, and going somewhere with lots of vegan options vs. somewhere with no vegan options can make all of the difference in the vegan world. For example: Italy and Greece are neighboring countries with similar cultures and are both very interesting, with lots of cool monuments and a lot to see and do. Food wise, Italy has lots of vegan options that include pizza and even soy ice cream shops, vs. Greece which has some Italian food, and rice wrapped in Grape Leaves (SGT VEGAN NOTE: Unless you go to Greece during Lent, which changes the experience completely). Making the choice to go to Italy vs. Greece will give you a completely different culinary experience if you are traveling, and can be the difference between vegan fun and epic failure.

2. Do your research. Researching your destination and having a list of vegan restaurants and places where you can go will make your trip more fun. Everybody loves food, and you

are going to be hard-pressed to find a country where you can't find any vegan restaurants. Do your research before you go, and have the vegan places you want to visit selected before you go. There are a lot of restaurant finder apps out there – one of the easiest to use is called "Happy Cow." Also, look up popular, easily veganized dishes from the countries you are headed to, because eating like the locals is often better than finding a vegan restaurant. Sometimes you will have to look outside the box to find good vegan options. For example: When traveling to Japan, you can easily find vegan food at any Kaiten Zushi (revolving sushi) restaurant, because most of the cheap items on the menu are vegan by default. Make sure you always do your vegan research. Remember, fortune favors the prepared vegan!

3. Bring your own food, within reason. If you are traveling within the USA on a road trip (hopefully a vegan one), bring a box of Cliff Bars and some fruit. That way, if you get hungry and aren't anywhere near a major city, you can easily eat and keep moving towards somewhere more vegan friendly. Also, there are some staples that are going to be harder to find, like vegan sausages, or vegan cheese, or vegan marshmallows; why not have them stashed? You will always be able to find more vegan spaghetti, noodles, or sauce, so don't even bother bringing them. Save the room in your car for the things you can't find anywhere else, and make sure they are stored in a well-insulated cooler.

4. Travel with like-minded, or at least vegan-friendly people. When it comes to being vegan, some people get it and some people don't. You don't need to travel exclusively with fellow vegans. However, if you are on a Vegan Road Trip, it is always going to be easier to travel with someone who understands why you want to go four hours out of your way for a vegan sticky bun, vs. someone who still thinks you are being a "picky eater" for not wanting to eat a carcass.

5. If you travel to another country, learn some of the language. I suck at learning languages, but when I travel I always learn a few phrases I can use here and there to get what I want. Sometimes just being able to say "hello" in the local language will be all you need to soften people up and get them to accommodate you. I have been to France, and while it wasn't the most vegan friendly place in the world, I didn't get the vibe of "French snobbery" Americans often complain about. It isn't that I "fit in"- SGT Vegan is as obviously American as Vegan Apple Pie. I think the reason why I didn't get snubbed in France is because I never assume people speak English when I travel. Whether it was French, Italian, Spanish, Japanese, Chinese, or even Arabic, I've always made the effort to speak some of the native language. No matter where you go people appreciate it. I don't blame the French for their disgust at the "American arrogance" for expecting the French to speak English while in their own country. That's as ridiculous as someone coming to my country, and expecting me to speak any other language but AMERICAN!!

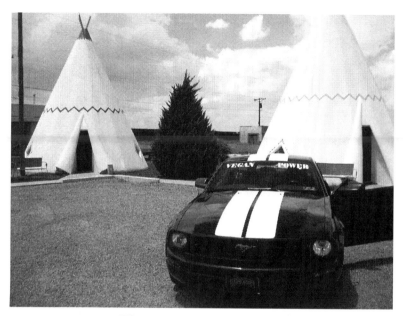

"Vegan Mobile 1 (Mustang)

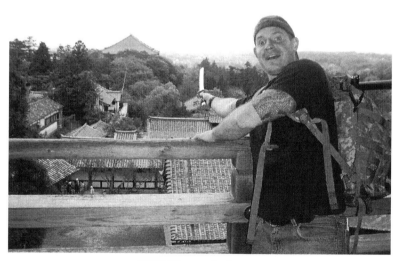

SGT Vegan in Japan

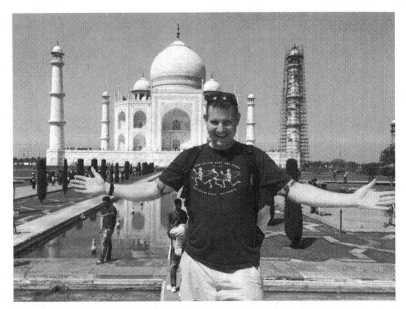

SGT Vegan in India

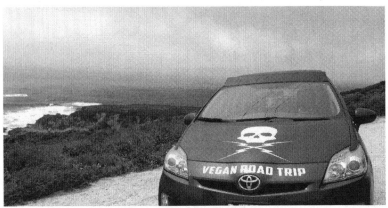

Vegan Mobile 2 (Prius)

Chapter 10

Dating in a Non-Vegan World

LET'S FACE IT: BEING VEGAN can make dating even more difficult than it already is. Trying to exclusively date vegans might be seen as limiting your romantic options. So, should you convert a meat-eater into being vegan, or only date people who have already made the decision to be vegan? Is it worth going through the hassle of dating a non-vegan with the hope that they turn vegan someday? In matters of the heart, you don't want to have to settle just so you won't have to eat your tofu burritos alone. Does it matter if your kids eat vegan, or if your spouse eats the same way as you do? There are indeed too many vegan questions and not enough answers.

In an effort to shed some light on the subject, I asked Dave Rubin from Veggie Date (www.veggiedate.org) to come talk to us about his website and to share some knowledge about dating, relationships, and being vegan.

Dave, please tell us about Veggie Date. How long have you been running the site, and what has the reception been like?

'VeggieDate' is one of the two largest vegetarian dating sites. VeggieDate was created in 1999 by Steve Urow. I started running VeggieDate in Sept. 2012. Hundreds of people have found their partner on VeggieDate.

Some facts about our members:

- Between 4,000 and 5,000 new members join each year.
- 63% of our visible members identify as "vegan", "raw" or "veggie/veganish" (39% vegan)
- 55% are men vs. 45% women.
- 8.1% identify as bisexual
- 3.3% identity as gay.
- 59% have a college degree (Associates or higher).
- 31% identify as something other than Caucasian

Some people meet partners, business associates or friends, on VeggieDate. It seems to me that those who live in cities where there is a relative concentration of vegans or vegetarians and/or who are willing to date outside their area are more likely to make a connection. We have been working on making the site friendly for mobile users and, we are nearly finished with that project. I am hopeful this and other things I am working on will help us to get to the next level. Some people have expressed appreciation for VeggieDate and for what I do. Some people do not like that we charge to initiate contact with another member, even though reading and responding to messages is free. I think some people do not realize that we do not have sufficient traffic to operate the site exclusively with advertising revenue. Overall, I would say the reception has been mostly positive.

How have your views on dating changed since you've been running the website?

I don't think running the website has changed my thinking. It seems to me that if a person who has vegan values wants to find a partner with similar values or co-parent while teaching vegan values to his or her children, it is essential to find a vegan partner. A vegetarian dating site can facilitate this.

Any weird/funny/standout profiles that are worth sharing?

In reading the profiles, it is clear to me that we have a diverse membership. Some have perspectives I easily connect with and resonate with and some have perspectives that do not resonate with me. I would like to invite the readers to check out the profiles for themselves and make their own judgments.

Any success stories from your dating site?

I personally know several couples who married after meeting on VeggieDate, including some leaders in the vegan community (Eric and Diana from Happy Cow, Allison and David from Allison's Gourmet, and Laura and Robert who are organizing SoCal VegFest in Orange County).

Advice for vegans?

I think finding a compatible partner (or partners if polyamorous) can really help a person to heal, grow, and move forward in creating what we want in life. If you identify as vegan, you may find that you have preferences regarding your partner's lifestyle. I think it can really help to provide peace, clarity, ease, and emotional safety for you and a potential partner to be really clear on what you want before you start a new relationship. If you are not yet clear on what you require in this regard, here are some questions to consider: What are the reasons you have chosen a vegan lifestyle? Is it important to you to have a partner who shares your core ethics and values? Do you plan to raise children with your partner? If yes, do you want to teach them vegan values? Are you comfortable kissing someone who might have recently eaten animal products? Are you comfortable having animal products in your home? Are you comfortable eating with a date or partner who is consuming animal products?

I think that becoming clear on who you want to invite into your life is a critical step. If you decide that having a partner who is committed to a vegan lifestyle is essential, you now have the challenge of finding a vegan partner. It seems to me that the vegan population has grown exponentially in the last couple of decades, so it is a lot easier than it once was to find a vegan partner. To improve your chances of finding a compatible partner, consider utilizing a variety of strategies such as putting your profile on the major vegetarian websites such as VeggieDate and Veggie Connection. Go to events where you will meet other vegans. Join and interact on Vegan Facebook groups. Let your friends introduce you to possible romantic interests, etc. It's my perspective that the more you do to increase your chances and invite what you want into your life, the more likely it is that you will get what you want.

Another thing to consider is whether or not you are willing to consider dating a non-vegan who you think might choose a vegan lifestyle once he or she connects with and understands the benefits. If yes, consider how close (in terms of physical intimacy, emotional connection, frequency of visits, etc.) you can get to someone before that person commits to a vegan lifestyle. How will you ensure that you do not get closer than you want to be? How will you know if that person is really committed to the lifestyle or is really motivated to get close to you?

Thank you, SGT Vegan for your interest and the opportunity to tell your readers about VeggieDate and to share my thoughts and perspectives."

Thank you for your wisdom and advice, Dave. Good luck everyone. Remember, vegan or not, love is a battlefield! Stay safe out there!

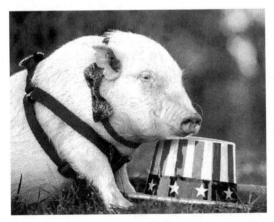

Freedom is love.

Photo Courtesy of Terran Vincent Baylor

Chapter 11

Vegan Activism 101

BY NOW IT SHOULD NOT come as a shock I believe we have to stop the animal slaughter industry. If you are still reading my words you might also be interested in becoming a part of this movement as well. What follows are some tips about activism, how to get started, and some thoughts on the whole matter. While this in no way is the "final word" on activism, I hope you will find these ideas are helpful to you.

1. Social media is a great place to see what's out there. You should join some online animal rights groups and see what is going on in your area and what you can do to help. You can also get in contact with like-minded people and make friends. Mainstream society calls this "Networking," but this is just as important in trying to change the world as it is in changing your job. It always helps to know people.

2. Check out animal right's organizations such as PETA/Mercy for Animal/Vegan Outreach. No, I don't agree with 100% of everything these organizations do in trying to get across the vegan message, but they are usually at least close to the target. These groups organize their own protests and you can be a part of them to get the feel for it. You can also get signs and flyers from them if you want to do your own thing, just by writing to them and requesting they send them to you.

3. I have heard some activists argue for a "by any means necessary" approach to ending the slaughter of animals. However, I will always argue AGAINST using violence to further Animal Rights no matter how slow progress may be. Most of us were not born vegan. Therefore, we too have been guilty, and should be wary of being too judgmental towards others. If we use violence, then we are (almost) as bad as what we are fighting against. I understand millions of innocent animals are dying while we slowly work at getting people to eat more veggie burgers. I understand direct action might seem more appealing than talking to people about why they should have Meatless Mondays (followed by every other day of the week as well). Still, bringing this common sense message to people is what is going to create real, lasting change. Being violent, whether in acts or words towards the people who disagree with us will only discredit the movement and be a further step back for the animals. So talk to a hunter and get him to agree to try some meat alternatives. Give a pamphlet to a shopper at Whole Foods. Do all of that but channel a little MLK as well, and do it with intelligence, professionalism, and a touch of class.

4. Practice t-shirt activism - wear your favorite vegan t-shirt to the gym. Nothing destroys myths about vegans being unhealthy like being more fit than those around you. Let your workout doing the talking for you.

5. Always remember when you talk to people about being vegan, you become a representative for the vegan lifestyle. You might be the first vegan someone has ever met, and a first impression is not just an important thing, it is everything! I'm not talking about hippy karma, positive vibes, and all of that "peace and love" stuff. No, I'm talking about effectively marketing being vegan in a way which will grow the animal rights movement and save more animals in the long run. We need to make people

WANT to be vegan, not turn them off to the idea of it. Think of using the soft sell: explain the reasons for being vegan, and give people the awesome reasons for making the switch, but don't be too self-righteous about it. The only thing that happens when we come off like jerks is we make it easier for people to close their minds to the truth. The seeds you plant in people's brains today will sprout someday if you give them a chance. Nurture those seeds with understanding and compassion because the kid you talk to today might someday lead the next generation of vegans.

6. There has been an unfortunate trend lately among so-called activists to focus negative attention on vegetarians for not going far enough with their commitment to animals to be vegan. Obviously it is better to be vegan than to be eating dairy and eggs for many reasons which we have already discussed, but to be angry at someone for not having enough "follow through" is completely unproductive and somewhat hypocritical. In order for this movement to keep going, we need to be inclusive and accept anyone and everyone who would help move the ball forward in this fight for a more compassionate world. Every person counts, and to alienate our allies only diminishes our numbers and weakens the movement's potential.

7. My new favorite activism tool is the screen projector. The screen projector is a big spotlight that can turn any wall into a billboard for your custom-made vegan sign. Best thing about it? It is perfectly legal as long as you are standing on public property (like a side walk) and not blocking any foot traffic (SGT VEGAN NOTE: Please do your own research about local and state laws). In the US it is protected by First Amendment freedom of speech laws, though you would probably be shut down if you add obscenities to your sign. With limited amount of searching on the Internet you can find out how to make your own

Vegan Spotlight so you can start enlightening the world today!

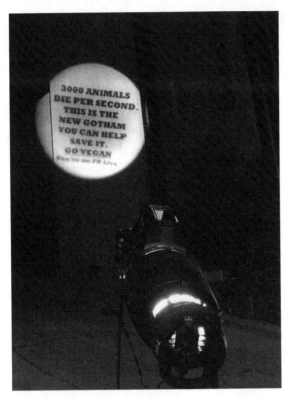

Shine a light on the injustice in the world

Chapter 12

Veganism and Punk Rock

I BECAME A VEGETARIAN at the age of 18 in the height of my punk rock years. I was a freshman in college, with an exciting new world of ideas opening before me. Being a punk rocker meant an opportunity for me to re-examine who I was, and to consciously rebuild myself. I found meaning in the lyrics of the short, angry songs of punk music. I studied sociology and politics and wanted to help end the oppression, racism, and sexism I saw inherent in modern society. I took to heart Mahatma Gandhi's saying, "Be the change you want to see in the world." I figured not eating animals was a great place to start making that change into a reality.

My journey in self-exploration began when I gave up drinking the first week of my freshman year in college. At a time when most people have their first beer, I had my last. The summer before college, I had worked on a ship as a deckhand (SGT VEGAN NOTE: I don't know how anyone can say the word "seaman" with a straight face. Sorry, Navy!). It was truly an eye-opening experience. I had a front-row seat to what alcoholism was and how it had ruined the lives of several of my fellow crew members. While that summer had started as an all out booze-fest, I saw the problems I could get into with drinking if I followed down the same path. I vowed alcohol would never ruin my life, and the thought stayed with me after I walked down the gangplank and into college life.

A band called Minor Threat gave words to what I was thinking with the song "Straight Edge," which championed mental freedom through substance-free living. I liked that they did not see this lifestyle as a "set of rules" to push on people, but rather about giving an alternative to mainstream culture's destructive "party" mentality. I realized I could be more of who I was and wanted to be if I stopped altering my mind. It wasn't about disliking people who drank; it was about doing my own thing and respecting the rights of others to do the same. People who thought this way were called Straight Edge, named after the song. I joined their ranks after I took my last sip of beer in my college dorm in September 1991.

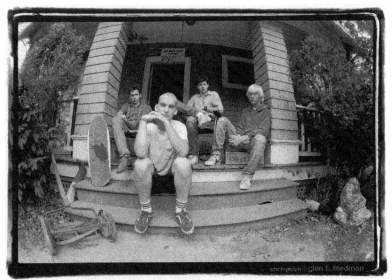

Minor Threat, photo courtesy of Glen E. Friedman.

I became vegetarian somewhat by accident. It was the winter of 1992 and my Mom had been asking me to give up something for Lent. To get her to stop bugging me, and because I wanted to push the Limits of the known Universe, I told her I was going to give up eating meat. I figured if the Catholics don't eat meat on Fridays during Lent, I can one-up them by not eating meat during the entire 40 days of Lent. While this would just be considered a trendy "cleanse" now, back in 1992 this was nothing short of revolutionary. People told me I was going to get sick, and friends and family sat back and waited for me to die. I remember someone actually telling me, "Nice knowing you." To be honest, I myself didn't know what was going to happen. At that point I wasn't doing it to save the animals or the planet. I stopped eating meat because I wanted to push boundaries and question "truths."

To the surprise of friends and family, instead of having to plan my funeral, they watched me get healthier. I got into better shape and even put on muscle. Being vegetarian wasn't all that difficult even back then, and I didn't give it much thought after the first couple of months. I was happily living in my own little bubble.

Up until the summer, I did not meet any other vegetarians, nor did I read anything on the subject. I was just doing my own thing. In the pre-Internet-days things were different than they are now. You still had to get information from books, not by "Googling it," and some knowledge had to be passed from person to person. The downside of this was if you didn't know the right people, you probably wouldn't get the right information. For example, I found out about gelatin at a party. Someone suggested we see how many marshmallows we could fit in our mouths at one time, and of course everyone did it because we were still dumb kids, even without any alcohol. Someone else remarked I was not a real vegetarian because I was eating marshmallows, which contained gelatin. I had no idea what gelatin was and searched the house for a dictionary. I couldn't believe the main ingredient in Jell-O and marshmallows came from boiling horse hoofs and assorted animal parts and then skimming off the slime. That was the last time I had a marshmallow until I had a vegan one made by Chicago Soy Dairy two decades later.

I also soon learned how cheese was made. That summer I drove my Volkswagen Dasher into the ground for $5 an hour plus mileage and tips delivering pizza (SGT VEGAN NOTE: Don't deliver pizza in an old stick shift car you care about). There never was much in the way of tips, and $5 an hour sucked even back then. Free pizza at work was a pretty good perk until I heard about rennet. Rennet is an enzyme taken from a baby cow's stomach and is used to make cheese. I'm sure there are a lot of rennet-free cheeses out there now, but at the time I stopped eating cheese, all of them seemed to contain it. Of course, to get the rennet to make cheese they had to kill the baby cow first. When I first stopped eating cheese, I was okay with pulling the cheese off the pizza, but the more I read, the less okay I was with animal products even touching my food. That's when I knew the big change was coming. The check was in the mail.

I had originally told myself I would only become a lacto/ovo vegetarian, but after some serious thought, I went vegan. (SGT VEGAN NOTE: Lacto/ovo are some fancy words people use to say they still eat eggs and drink milk.) The decision was easy because the question was simple. The time had come when I had to decide once and for all exactly how much animal abuse I was ok with. I wasn't ok with eating the bodies of dead animals, so why was I ok with having animals die so I could eat cheese or drink milk? Did I really want to support the industries that enslave and kill animals just so I wouldn't be inconvenienced?

Being Vegan Straight Edge was still seen as something very radical, which reinforced my punk rock identity and made it feel like the right thing to do. Punk rock was always about following your heart, so I didn't care if it was unpopular. I started to see a parallel between society's addiction to drugs and alcohol and an obsession with killing animals for food. I used to buy the line we needed to eat animals for health reasons, but then again I used to believe you had to drink alcohol to have fun. Here I was, totally happy and healthy with no animals in my stomach or alcohol in my blood. Obviously mainstream knowledge had gotten it all wrong once again.

It was exciting to follow bands that were writing songs about things that mattered, unlike most of the pop music of the day. I got into Bad Brains, Fugazi, Slapshot, Public Enemy, and of course, Rage Against the Machine. I wanted the music I was consuming to echo some part of my new-found consciousness. Then I heard about some bands that specifically promoted an animal rights message. Two NYC bands stood out. Youth of Today had a song called "No More," about going Meat Free, and Gorilla Biscuits had a song called "Cats and Dogs," about how we pet dogs and cats while we kill cows and pigs. There was also the British ska band called Citizen Fish (formerly the Subhumans) that had numerous songs about Animal Rights.

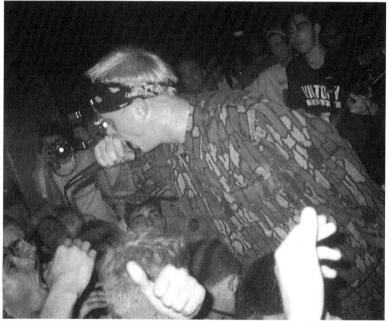

Earth Crisis circa 1996, photo courtesy of Brian X Suhr.

Then along came the band Earth Crisis, and everything changed. Earth Crisis wrote metal songs with lyrics about animal slaughter and saving the planet. They started as an underground band with zero commercial appeal, but they went on to play the OZZFEST (Ozzy Osborne's travelling metal music festival), had a video on MTV, and toured the world. For a couple of years, they were confronting, educating, and pissing-off people at shows all around the world with their militant stance. Love them or hate them, Earth Crisis helped bring Animal Rights Awareness to the mainstream.

Writing this many years later, still young at heart but on the verge of middle age, I look back and smile when I think about punk rock and the time in my life it represents. Similar to the folk protest bands of the 1960's, punk rock was more than just music; it was about changing the world. Growing up on the East Coast, the only activists I knew were either punk rockers or holdouts from the hippy era, and there was a certain camaraderie in that small community. It felt like it was just us against the world, screaming for change. Unfortunately, an unintentional side effect of that camaraderie was we made being vegan into an exclusive secret club which only let members of the fringe inside.

While there may be some who want to keep our movement a secret club, I'm excited veganism has spread into the mainstream. We need to share this with every person on the planet, not keep it to ourselves! I'm always happy when I meet "normal" people --yogis, lawyers, athletes, businessmen, students, and others-- who agree eating vegan is better for the planet, our health, and the animals. I've been working for the government for a couple of years now, and while I don't look the part of the punk rocker anymore, the message remains the same. Go Vegan and together we can change the world, one meal at a time!

Toby Morse

Singer in punk band H2O

How long have you been vegan?

I have been vegan since 1989.

How/why did you go vegan and why are you still vegan?

I saw the PETA videos when I was 18 yrs old. The punk scene in NYC at the time, specifically the straightedge movement, had Krishna influences. Vegan and vegetarian consciousness really connected to me.

How has being vegan changed your life?

I don't feel my age at all. I'm still doing what I did as a kid - skating, exercising etc. My son has been raised vegetarian his whole life. He's 14 and never had meat. Our whole family is cruelty free!

Tell me about something cool that you've done.

I became a father.

Advice for new vegans?

Don't preach it too much. You're doing it for the animals and the planet. When you preach it to people, it turns them off. Teach it; don't preach it.

Favorite restaurant?

Crossroads (Los Angeles, CA)

Chapter 13

The Vegan Guide to the Zombie Apocalypse

PEOPLE SOMETIMES ASK ME if I would remain vegan during a variety of absurd circumstances. The important question to ask should not be if I would remain vegan during the Zombie Apocalypse, but why people still choose to eat dead animals in the 21st century when there are so many delicious, cruelty-free vegan foods available! As you may already know, zombies are science fiction. The chances of a Zombie Apocalypse happening are about as likely as the chances of meeting an honest politician. So while we can safely rule out an Apocalypse with actual Zombies, we could consider it as a metaphor for a momentary breakdown of society. Think of it this way: during the last thirty years, the US has had numerous crises where being prepared would have made the difference between life and death, whether Katrina in New Orleans, tornados in the Midwest, hurricanes and other storms in NJ and FL, riots and unrest on both coasts, and earthquakes in LA. Will America be here forever? The smart money says no. Just like Rome, we too will someday fall, but HOPEFULLY NOT anytime in the near future. Like it or not, though, society will unravel a little every now and then. While I was in Afghanistan, I watched a news report about the people in Louisiana affected by the flooding during Hurricane Katrina. I remember thinking, "Damn, those people have it rough." Bad things can happen anywhere, at any time, and it always is good to be prepared and have a plan. While this all may seem ridiculous to consider, the fact remains that in life there are some extraordinary scenarios when the unexpected happens and an ounce of preparation is worth a pound of gold. Remember, fortune favors the prepared vegan!

The following is a common sense packing list to help you stay alive and vegan during the Zombie Apocalypse. While I personally don't own a working firearm and support laws to keep guns out of the wrong hands, I couldn't write a chapter about the Zombie Apocalypse without mentioning them. Good Luck! You'll need it!

1. Have a good stash of water. You can't live without water for longer than a few days to a week. It can cost a lot of money and make you look like a crazy "doomsday prepper" if you build a bunker in your backyard. However, having enough water to last you a week is not only a cheap way of being prepared, it is also the most important thing you can do to be ready for anything, and won't make you look like a weirdo.

2. Having a good stash of food should already be common sense for the vegan. If good vegan food is sometimes hard to come by now, it will be crazy impossible to find when disaster strikes. Remember, the rest of the people around you won't be so picky, so you especially need to be ready for this. I suggest a mix of durable food items, such as canned foods (don't forget the can-opener), ramen noodles (not the cup type, a waste of money, and read the ingredients before you buy), Cliff Bars or other protein bars, and some shelf-stable soy/rice milk. Make sure you have a camp stove to cook the noodles (with extra propane cans), or some MRE heaters. Remember you will probably lose electricity, so perishable items and frozen foods will spoil. Eat them first in the event of a catastrophe, and save

the durable goods for later. Trail mix and raisins are a good idea for shelf-stable energy.

3. Flashlights, blankets, sleeping bag. You aren't going to be able to rely on the gas company to heat your house, and it's going to get cold. Also, you are going to need a source of light. Have plenty of batteries stocked.

4. Practical, durable clothes. In 21ˢᵗ Century America the majority of people I see everyday do not wear clothes with any practical value to them. By this I mean they wear clothes they can't run or fight in and won't protect them from the elements. I'm also guilty of this, because unless I am going to work, I often dress like I'm headed to the beach. Women are told by society they should dress "sexy", which usually means shoes a person couldn't comfortably walk in and clothes that restrict movement. When people get home from work, they are used to dressing as if they are headed to the sofa to binge watch a show on Netflix. This is especially evident in Southern California, where it doesn't often rain, and most days are 70 degrees and sunny. At bare minimum, practical clothing means not only something you could wear to the gym and workout in, but also protect you from the elements if need be. Being prepared means having sensible shoes, preferably ones that are waterproof, because nothing ends a good day like a pair of wet socks. A good jacket (also waterproof) is worth its weight in gold.

5. Weapon? To weapon or not to weapon, that is the question. I don't own a firearm (unless you count the one hanging on my wall from the 1800's that they no longer make bullets for), and support strict gun laws and a rethinking of the second amendment, but in the case of the apocalypse, a firearm would definitely be useful. The pistol has its advantages as it is easily concealable and portable, but lacks range and stopping power. The rifle has the range the pistol lacks but might take a little bit of time to learn

how to use. The shotgun takes less time getting used to, has less magazine capacity than either the pistol or rifle, but has more stopping power than either and will scare the average bad guy when you pump it. Whichever way you go with a firearm, make sure you know what you are doing with it, or it will easily be turned on you. Also, take your body size into consideration. Male or female, a 90 lb. person is too small for a hand cannon like a .44 magnum, and a shotgun will knock your shoulder off. Take a weapons class, don't point your weapon at anyone you don't plan to kill, and always treat every gun like it's loaded. If you do have to shoot someone other than a zombie, don't waste your time with a headshot. The head is a small target, and hard to hit. Instead, take your time, and place two well-aimed shots in the center of the chest of the person that means you harm. In the old days we used to call that the "double tap", but now it is called a "controlled pair" in this kinder and gentler era. Remember, bullets will be hard to come by in a time of crisis, and a good knife or baseball bat will be an important tool to have in threat-elimination.

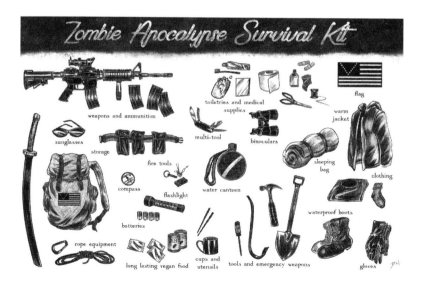

Part 2

VEGAN POWER

Chapter 14

Vegan Nutrition

As an RN working in a Cardiac Ward, the subject of nutrition is near and dear to my heart (pun intended). I work with patients every day who are suffering from a variety of self-inflicted ailments (from obesity to cardiac and pulmonary issues), many of which could be treated with a change in eating habits. Of course, change is difficult, and many people would rather take medication than change their lifestyle. Still, I firmly believe that until you are dead and in the ground you can always change your life for the better.

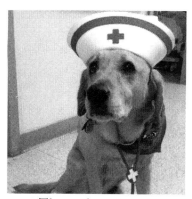

The author at work

Before I start talking about healthy eating, I would like to say that the most obvious positive lifestyle choice someone can make is to NOT smoke anything. I say "anything" because while people usually agree with not smoking cigarettes or crack, they always ask "what about vaping or smoking marijuana?" Here's the deal: smoking cigarettes has been positively linked to causing lung cancer. No one is debating this fact, and I'm not even going to cite evidence because I shouldn't have to convince you of this, any more than I should have to back up the earth being round or that climate change is affecting our world. We don't really know about E-cigs or marijuana yet, but the current best medical guess is while they might not be as harmful as regular cigarettes, they should by no means be considered "healthy".

Doctors used to think smoking was good for you and even endorsed certain cigarette brands, so don't take the current lack of information from the medical community as a green light to use them. These smoking alternatives can still cause irritation to the bronchial lining, and there may be other risks as well to using them that we don't know of because the research isn't in yet. In short, while e-cigarettes and marijuana might be a safer to smoke than tobacco products, try to avoid long-term use. (SGT VEGAN NOTE: For some information, please check out the American Lung Association homepage, www.lung.org)

In addition, you don't have to be Straight Edge to realize drinking a case of beer a day isn't good for you either. I have seen enough patients with liver damage to know excessive drinking can and will damage the liver, and without the liver (the body's filter) you are in trouble. So please approach alcohol with moderation. As for harder drugs, if you want to see some unhealthy people, talk to someone who uses meth or heroin. Please stay away from these drugs, and if you use them, concentrate on conquering that addiction first before you even consider trying to change your diet. You can only climb one mountain at a time.

So on to food, glorious food. In America too many of us "live to eat" when we should be "eating to live." I am not arguing we shouldn't be enjoying what we are eating. I am just saying there are healthier, cruelty-free foods we should be eating instead. I don't believe we need to give up all sugar and deprive ourselves like monks or to go "full hippy" with juice fasts. The trick to eating healthy is not a trick. It is a common sense set of guidelines which are easy to follow for the rest of your life, not about a quickie diet for a couple of weeks. Take a look at our obesity epidemic if you have any doubt Americans are having a hard time figuring out what to put in their mouths. Be not afraid, America! SGT Vegan is here to lead you out of the darkness and into the light of healthy eating.

Let us first understand that the calorie is the basic unit of energy your body needs to sustain life. Think of a calorie like gasoline for your car. Not enough gas and your car runs out of fuel, and then you are stuck without a Super WAWA in sight (SGT VEGAN NOTE: For those not from the American East Coast, WAWA is the best convenience store on earth). Too many calories in your system is like filling up your gas tank and then pouring the rest of the gas all over your car and in your back seat. It is a sloppy, dangerous mess that is sure to explode and end in death.

The answer to how many calories your body needs every day is around 2000 for the average woman, and around 2500 for the average male. This number varies depending on your age, body type, gender, and lifestyle. Women generally tend to need fewer calories than men, unless they are pregnant, exercising heavily, or healing due to an illness. Those times in life require more calories, more fuel to feed the body as it heals itself. People who are trying to put on muscle need more calories as well to build themselves up. Remember, unused calories will be stored as fat, and extra calories every day will lead to extra pounds over time.

There are a couple of different ways to figure out how much you are eating. If you are my Mom, you inventory everything you eat and count your calories using measuring cups, a scale, and a calorie book. That takes a lot of time and discipline but is incredibly effective. Though my mom is in her 70s, she still weighs around the same as she did in high school and hasn't had to deal with the cancer, heart disease, or diabetes that has plagued her side of the family. She does this by watching what she eats and exercising daily. Even though my mom still eats meat she always makes vegetables the main attraction of every meal. This is very similar to the Japanese way of eating. As a people, the Japanese are slim without the widespread use of gyms, because they generally walk or ride bikes daily and eat in moderation.

Remember, extra calories your body doesn't need will be stored as fat, and empty calories (calories with no nutritional value) are empty calories whether they are vegan or not. I think it is important to note that just because something is vegan doesn't necessarily make it a healthy food choice. Oreos might now be technically vegan (the debate over palm oil aside), but they can't be considered a healthy food. I am vegan and can tell you a million reasons why you shouldn't eat a fish, but I wouldn't be a good RN if I told you that eating Oreos is better for your health than eating fish. Being vegan IS much healthier than the Standard American Diet IF DONE PROPERLY, so let's always aim to eat healthy, vegan meals, and avoid junk foods.

Alternatively, I have some very healthy non-vegan friends who eat right and exercise every day. They are people who live the basic nutrition tips I am imparting to you, but they still eat meat occasionally. So please don't ASSUME just because something is vegan it is always going to be healthier, or that just because something is animal-based it will inherently be super unhealthy. As vegans we must always spread the TRUTH, not blind PROPAGANDA. Remember, there are three main reasons people are vegan, but everyone comes to Veganville of their own free will and on their own terms.

While my Mom's approach of calorie counting definitely works, most people don't have the time to write down everything they eat. I know I don't. As an RN, I work 12-hour shifts, and often I don't have enough time to pee, let alone count up everything I eat down to the last calorie. What follows is some basic nutrition advice. Keep in mind a diet derived from a variety of sources and rich in all food groups (other than animal sources) will be better than a diet coming from only one source. So go ahead, eat a big salad, and pile on the vegetables and whole grains, but just take it easy on the fatty heavily caloric salad dressings and sauces. Eat carbohydrates and give your body the energy it needs, but stay away from simple sugars like candy, as they are empty calories. Take it easy when it comes to fats, but scarf down that handful of almonds in your Silk Yogurt you are having for your snack at work. In other words, other than the part where your parents told you that you needed to eat meat and drink milk to grow big and strong, you should follow the same nutrition advice your parents gave you as a kid that you straight-up ignored.

As we have discussed, people need around 2000-2500 calories a day to maintain their current body requirements of life (breathing, heart, body temperature regulation, etc.). That number is called the Resting Energy Expenditure (REE). If you Google "REE," there are a couple of websites that will work it all out for you, but if you want to go DIY here is one, thanks to *The US Navy SEAL Guide to Fitness and Nutrition*.[31]

Age	Equation to get REE
18-30	6.95x weight (in lbs.) +679
30-60	5.27x weight (in lbs.) + 879

So for *me*:

45 years old 193 lbs. male.   5.27 x 193 + 879 = 1896.11 calories needed to maintain my current body weight. Less calories means I lose weight; more calories mean I gain weight.

From there you estimate your level of activity.[32]

Level of Activity	Activity Factor
Very light – watching TV	1.3
Light- walking	1.6
Moderate-Jogging	1.7
Heavy-running a race	2.1
Super Crazy – like marathons	2.4

So for me, a 45-year-old 193- lb. male with a moderate exercise lifestyle (I lift weights almost every day but I am not going crazy) the equation I would use is 1896.11 x 1.7. That means I would need 3,223.387 calories to maintain my current body weight while working out a moderate amount, like going to the gym for an hour and a half or so and being on my feet most of the day. On days I sit and binge watch Netflix, the number is going to be far less, like 2464.9 calories. These charts are best used only as an estimate, but the concept is sound. On days when you burn a bunch of calories, you are going to need to replenish them or you are going to get weak from not having enough gas in the tank. If you are taking it easy and not working out, you are also going to have to take it easy on the fork as well, or your waistline is going to expand. Calories in vs calories out is a very simplistic but effective and scientific way to view eating and body weight.

The magic number of calories needed to gain or lose a pound of body weight is 3500.[33] That means one little extra cookie here and there means nothing by itself, but little things add up. Let's say you go to Starbucks everyday, and your latte is 100 calories. Does it matter if you drink one latte? No. But let's look at it over 1 year:

100 calories (actually much more, but to make the math work out easier let's stick with 100) x 365 days = 36500 calories extra. 365,000/3500 = 10 lbs. gained in 1 year due to lattes.

Verdict? Make your coffee at home, save the money, and don't gain 10 lbs. Weight gain during an injury, pregnancy, or a deployment is understandable and unavoidable. Extra flab on your tummy because you drink a latte every day is not only physically unappealing, but can also be unhealthy. (SGT VEGAN NOTE: While we are on the subject of lattes, it makes no sense to have to pay extra for cruelty-free milk at chains like that. Just say no to "vegan exploitation.")

Macronutrients

Let's move on to discussing our body's 3 main sources of energy: Carbohydrates (or CARBS for short), FAT, PROTEIN (or PRO for short).

<u>CARBS</u>

Carbohydrates have gotten a bad reputation lately, but don't believe the hype! Carbs are the main source of energy for humans. There are two types of carbs: simple and complex. Simple carbs (sugar, fructose from fruit, corn syrup) will give you a small burst of energy, but will quickly dissipate and leave your body wanting more. That is not to say eating a piece of fruit and a candy bar is the same. While a candy bar only contains empty calories, fruit contains fiber that is needed to keep you regular and make you feel full after a meal, as well as a plethora of essential vitamins. Complex carbs are found in grains, seeds, pasta, macaroni, beans, and all other vegetables, and are converted by the body into glucose to fuel the body. Complex carbs are the super fuel that will keep our bodies moving all day and keep our bodies and minds working soundly.

In terms of calories, 1 gram of CARBS = 4 calories, and we are going to want to get between 65- 80% of our calories from complex carbohydrates such as brown rice and quinoa, as well as fruit and vegetables which are full of fiber. In terms of a daily diet of 2000 calories, that would be 2000 x 80% = 1600 calories. Please read my words carefully: SGT Vegan did not just say to eat 1600 calories worth of cookies. No I did not! I am saying you should derive a majority of your calories from the COMPLEX CARBS you need for energy, and they should come from a variety of plant and fruit sources. Candy, sweets, and foods made from processed flours and refined sugars should ALWAYS be kept to a minimum.

People have been avoiding carbs lately because a man named "Dr." Atkins pandered to the discipline-adverse American public. His mantra? Eat all the meat and unhealthy food you want, just avoid the carbs and you will lose weight. In 2003 Atkins died, and the details surrounding his death are murky at best.[34] Many doctors have wondered if Atkins' own diet may have contributed to the heart problems that led to his death. Atkins's people maintain that the doctor slipped on some ice, hit his head, and died. Did his diet kill him in the end? I don't think it helped him stay healthy, that's for sure. Diets high in saturated fats like his have greater instances of heart disease, and it sounds like that was a contributing factor in his death. The Atkins diet does work in a way, though. People on that diet usually are at a loss as to what to eat because most things have carbs in them. This makes them eat less. Eating less will lead to weight loss, as we have seen. Making up for the lack of carbs with extra saturated fat will probably give you a heart attack so buyer beware.

So generally, when it comes to carbs I say eat them – but go for complex carbs like multi -grained bread, rice, and pasta, and fruits and vegetables. Fuel your body with lasting energy. Stay away from candy and simple carbs high in sugars. As far as High Fructose Corn Syrup goes, most studies I have seen report it isn't any worse for you than regular sugar.[35] That said, it appears in far too many products and shows up where it isn't wanted or even needed, and simple sugars aren't good for you either.

Extra sugar adds empty calories which leads to extra pounds, and a high sugar diet will also lead to tooth decay and type 2 diabetes. Take this seriously, because both of these WILL MESS YOU UP! Untreated type 2 diabetes-- the type of diabetes that is a result of poor lifestyle choices (bad food and not enough exercise) -- can lead to tissue death, diabetic foot ulcers, and the eventual amputation of your toes, feet, and even your legs!

As for your teeth, take care of them! Brush your teeth at least twice a day. I read somewhere the condition of your teeth is a good indication of your longevity. I feel the patients I see who are in overall good shape usually have good teeth, and the ones who look like a train wreck almost always have poor dentation (bad teeth), as well as copious other medical issues. While it is unclear if people's medical problems are caused by their poor dentation or if their poor dentation is a result of not caring about their health in general, there does seem to be a link between the two.

I am not going to brag, but SGT Vegan has never had a cavity. What is my secret? Well, three things: 1. I brush my teeth twice a day 2. Genetics and 3. I avoid sugary soda. Remember, I said avoid, not "don't drink at all." One soda every couple weeks is probably okay. One soda every day sucks. The little things you do or don't do every day (or most days) to improve your health pay dividends when you get older.

I am not saying you should never eat sugary snacks, have a piece of cake, or eat an Oreo cookie. I am saying there are many of vegan snacks that are not good for you even though they are vegan. In small quantities and every now and again it isn't a big deal, but in bigger quantities over time they will be problematic. You don't need to count calories when it comes to eating vegetables, but watch it with the heavily processed, empty calorie crap.

Lastly, let's talk about aspartame. The fans of aspartame say because it is 200 times sweeter than sugar it can add a sweet taste to food without adding calories. The detractors say it can cause Alzheimer's and headaches. After some research, it appears aspartame is generally safe for use,[36] but may trigger migraines in some people,[37] and depression in others.[38] If you have a medical condition called phenylketonuria, aspartame is NOT SAFE FOR CONSUMPTION,[39] though that can be similar to how wheat is safe for everyone who doesn't have Celiac's disease. SGT Vegan's medical advice? Don't drink soda every day, diet or otherwise. While regular soda will rot your teeth and make you fat for sure, I would also limit your chugging of diet soda as well. Moderation is always a good plan when it comes to most things in life. Please keep in mind that in the past, doctors endorsed cocaine-laced Coke-a-cola as a "pick me up" energy drink and used to be paid to peddle cigarettes as well. So like almost everything in life this information is subject to change.

FAT

Low fat was the diet of choice for years, and for good reasons. One gram of fat contains nine calories, so gram for gram it is a more energy-dense way to get calories. If you were a cave man ten thousand years ago, or are currently living in the frozen tundra, you might want to get a lot of your calories from fat. For the rest of us, extra fat results in extra calories which results in extra body weight. That is not to say we don't need a certain percentage of calories from fat. Fat helps keep the body insulated and protects the organs, helps on a cellular level to move nutrients throughout the body and build cell walls, and it keeps you warm and helps you float. Not enough of it is unhealthy, but too much of it will lead to heart disease and obesity, cancer, and diabetes.

What is a healthy amount of daily fat? SGT Vegan thinks that you should strive to get 10% of your daily calories from healthy fat. If you were getting about 10% of your dietary calories a day from fat, that would mean given a 2000 calories-a- day diet (2000x10%= 200 calories, 200/9) you would be eating 22.2 grams of fat. Remember fat is a very dense source of energy, so if you are stuck out in the tundra in the winter, and want to survive, reach for some fat. However, in the South Bay of Los Angeles with an average temperature of 65 degrees Fahrenheit and sunny where I am trying to see my abs, I will continue to limit my fat consumption.

I like to use cooking sprays instead of oil, which add only a small amount of fat to the food I cook. I also try to limit the amount of vegan butter (Earth Balance) that I put on my bagel or English muffin in the morning, or the scoops of ice cream that go in my mouth. When cooking with oil, reach for olive oil, but be mindful that one tablespoon of it contains 120 calories. Stay away from hydrogenated oils, and consider the amount of saturated fats you are eating.

Though we have been mostly talking about limiting our consumption of fat, consider some healthy sources of fat we should all have in our lives. As I said before, if you are cooking with oil, make sure it is olive oil. Throw that avocado on your sandwich for some healthy richly-flavored goodness; it will be worth the calories. While snacking, reach for a handful of nuts or seeds, like walnuts, peanuts, almonds, cashews, you will be happy you did. Avoid empty calories from fat sources, processed foods, cookies, and especially from Vegan Donuts (SGT VEGAN NOTE: I still love you, Vegan Treats!). Deep-fried foods, including French fries, should also be eaten only in moderation.

PROTEIN

Once you go vegan, people will start to ask you all of the time where you get your protein. It's ironic, because with all of the diet-related health issues in this country, from obesity to diabetes, somehow people have been duped into micro-focusing attention on the one thing that isn't a widespread problem here. In general, Americans need to eat more fiber, more salad, and more vegetables, but our diets are NOT lacking protein. If anything, we are actually eating too much protein. Remember, too much of a good thing does not necessarily mean a better thing!

We should derive between 10-20% of our daily caloric intake from Protein (PRO). This is based on the US Recommended Daily Allowance (RDA) of 10%, with special consideration for life situations. In cases where you are trying to pack on massive amounts of weight or muscle, sick, or pregnant, raise that number up to 20%. If we assume an average of around 2000 calories per day, that is 2000 x 10% = 200 calories from protein on average. Two hundred calories divided by four calories per gram means you want to eat about 50 grams of protein in a normal day. Keep in mind that according to *The China Study* your actual protein requirement is far lower, around 5-6%.[40] To hit either the RDA or *The China Study* recommended protein minimum shouldn't be any problem at all. Given that one serving of farfalle pasta from Trader Joe's has 7 grams of protein per serving (x2 servings as my portion would be), that's 14 grams right there. The average Veggie Burger has about 12 grams in it, but after the bun you are at about 17grams. Tofu has about 10 grams per serving, but combined with broccoli – see my recipe in the Vegan-Delicious chapter- you will be eating about 15 grams in a serving. A cup of quinoa, which normally doesn't even get mentioned as a protein, has 6 grams per cup. Of course there are also peanut butter, lentils and beans, which are great sources as well.

Unfortunately, more protein in your mouth does not necessarily equate to more muscle in your body. Please consider your body can only process up to 30 g of protein at a time, so if you are eating more than that at a time, you are just going to pee it out. What excess protein means in your diet is just more work for your kidneys to excrete the waste.[41] If you have ever worked with people in kidney failure who are going to dialysis once a week because their kidneys don't work anymore, you know that is not a road you want to go down. Play it safe when it comes to protein!

My suggestion for protein if you are trying to build muscle is to time your protein intake to coincide with your workout schedule. After I lift weights, I like to get a high protein meal or protein supplement in my system (like a Cliff Builder Bar) of about 20 grams of PRO within one hour after working out to give my body the protein it needs to rebuild itself. You don't need to get 20-30 grams of protein in addition to what you are already eating, just make that a part of your total daily protein intake.

Lastly, a word about complete versus non complete proteins. Surprise! All plant proteins are complete proteins. The animal agriculture industry pulled one over on us for years, getting vegans to "mix and match" our proteins to get all of the essential amino acids. None of that is necessary, although a diet coming from a wide variety of plant sources will be more fun and probably contain more vitamins and minerals in it as well.

Micronutrients – Vitamins and Minerals

Micronutrients are essential for our body to function in so many ways. They are called micronutrients because we only need a small amount of them every day, but the small amounts we need are vital to our health. Most of these can be obtained from eating a healthy, balanced diet, and some might be better obtained through dietary supplements. Remember, you only need 100% of your RDA of vitamins and minerals. Once you get 100%, whether through the food you are eating, or through supplements, getting more does not help you. In most cases you will pee out the excess, and in other cases getting too much of a good thing can actually be really bad for you.

VITAMINS

There are two main types of Vitamins: water-soluble and fat-soluble. Excess water-soluble vitamins are excreted through the urine when you go over your RDA allowance, and excess fat-soluble vitamins are stored in your fat. The way I learned to remember the difference between the two in nursing school is to use these two mnemonic devices: "Sea Bees" and "A Deck of Cheese."

WATER SOLUBLE VITAMINS

Sea Bees. "C B's." The Sea Bees were a part of the Navy that was responsible for construction. You think water when you think about the Navy. Vitamin C and all of the B vitamins are water soluble, so you will pee out what you don't need.

Vitamin C is a powerful antioxidant. An antioxidant is a molecule that stops the process of oxidation, which has been linked to cancer and diseases. In Vitamin C's case, it helps in the repair of connective tissues and bone and the resistance to infection and supports the immune system. It also protects you from scurvy, which should be of great concern to you if you are a pirate or are in the Navy. Vitamin C is found in fruits like oranges and apples, but did you know it is also in carrots and a lot of other vegetables? RDA for men is 90 mg and 75mg for women.[42]

Vitamin B1 (thiamin) is important for CARB metabolism and energy production, and supports heart and muscle function. The RDA for men is 1.2 mg, and 1.1 mg for women.[43] As an important note, as an RN, I often have to give alcoholics extra doses of B1, because alcohol interferes with the absorption of B1 and the lack of it can cause a disease called Beriberi, which is "beriberi" bad for you! Look that up if you are in doubt![44] You can get thiamin from enriched breads, grains, legumes and peas, nuts and seeds.

Vitamin B2 (riboflavin) is needed to do pretty much the same things as B1. The lack of it will cause stomatitis (inflammation of the mouth), in addition to feeling lethargic. For us vegans, it is sourced from green, leafy vegetables, nuts, and legumes. RDA for men is 1.3 mg, 1.1 mg for women.[45]

Vitamin B3 (niacin) is also used for energy production, but it is also important for fat and protein metabolism, and aerobic (including oxygen) metabolism. Vegan sources include peanuts, mushrooms, peas, seeds, and avocado. People often take niacin as a way to lower their cholesterol levels. Not enough niacin will result in a condition called pellagra, which is characterized by diarrhea, dementia, and death if left untreated. (SGT VEGAN NOTE: Before companies developed Statin drugs to lower cholesterol levels, they prescribed niacin. Don't go above the upper limit for this vitamin, as it can be toxic in high quantities.) The RDA for men is 16 mg, and 14 mg for women, with an upper limit of 35 mg daily.[46]

Vitamin B5 (pantothenic acid) is also essential for energy production from CARBS and fats, proper cell maintenance, and healthy skin. It is used to treat everything from alcoholism to baldness, and it can be applied topically to treat skin conditions. According to *Becoming Vegan*,[47] all plant foods have Vitamin B5 in them, and men and women both need 5 mg a day of it.

Vitamin B6 (pyridoxine) is really important for a lot of reasons. It is essential in energy synthesis, and is used in metabolizing protein, and in immune function. It also supports Red Blood Cell (RBC) production and helps prevent carpal tunnel by keeping joints and connective tissues healthy. *Becoming Vegan*[48] states that both men and women need between 1.3 – 1.7 mg of vitamin B6, and that some sources include bananas, nutritional yeast, whole grain products, soymilk and soy foods, and potatoes. Vitamin B6 deficiency is rare, and if you have it, take a B vitamin complex or a multivitamin!

Vitamin B12 (cobalamin) is required for the functioning of the brain and nervous system and RBC synthesis. B12 promotes energy production and growth. B12 is created by bacterial symbiosis, and is found in the soil. Unfortunately, since we usually clean our veggies so well most of is washed off. Not having enough B12 WILL MESS YOU UP, eventually even causing severe damage to the brain and nervous system. I think it is better to be on the safe side and take a daily multivitamin for this one. There are a lot of foods that have added B12 to them, like some brands of nutritional yeast, and soy milk. For example, 8 oz. of the Chocolate Silk I am drinking as I write this (yum) has 50% of the RDA of B12. (SGT VEGAN NOTE: Silk isn't giving me a dime to say this, but I really like their soy milk.) The amount of B12 you need to prevent problems is relatively small. Per *Becoming Vegan*[49], we need between 2.4 - 2.8 micrograms per day for both men and women, and most cases of deficiency are due to poor absorption.

FAT SOLUBLE VITAMINS

A deck of cheese. "ADEK of cheese." A deck of cards is about the size of a block of cheese. No, you shouldn't be eating animal cheese, but when you think cheese, you think fat, so this mnemonic device should help you remember these fat-soluble vitamins. Vitamins A, D, E, and K are fat soluble, which means they are absorbed with dietary fat and stored in the tissues. You need these vitamins in your life, but unlike the water- soluble vitamins, if you take in too much of these by accident, they will MESS YOU UP!! So watch out. The American Way of thinking - if a little is good a lot must be great - DOES NOT APPLY HERE! Please stick with the daily recommended doses of these vitamins!

Vitamin A is a powerful antioxidant. It supports the immune system, protects the skin from the sun's ultraviolet damage, and the lungs from pollutants, and is important in making proteins in tendons and bones. In healthy people, Beta Carotene becomes Vitamin A and does the same thing. Some sources of Vitamin A include spinach and carrots, and most orange-colored vegetables. RDA is 800 mcg for women and 1000 micrograms for men. Don't go too far above that, supplemented Vitamin A will be harmful if taken above RDA amount.[50]

Vitamin D regulates the metabolism of calcium, which you need for healthy bones. Your body naturally produces Vitamin D when exposed to the sun. This doesn't mean you need to go get a tan to get some Vitamin D; only 20 minutes of being in the sun a day will get the job done. If you spend twelve hours a day indoors like me, that might be difficult, in which case you should either eat a lot of mushrooms (shiitake or portabella, which are great sources), or eat Vitamin D fortified foods, which are abundant these days. (SGT VEGAN NOTE: Watch out for Vitamin D3, which is usually animal-sourced. Vitamin D 2 is fine.) *Becoming Vegan* recommends between 5-15 micrograms a day,[51] which you should be careful to get if you don't get out to see the sun often or are a vampire night worker like me.

Vitamin E is an antioxidant important for immune function. Some sources for Vitamin E include wheat germ, olive oil, whole grains, and leafy green vegetables like spinach. Per Becoming *Vegan* the RDA for adults of Vitamin E is 15 mg.[52] Be careful because too much Vitamin E can put you at a greater risk for bleeding, so take it easy on the supplements!

Vitamin K assists in blood clotting, and can be found in green, leafy vegetables, broccoli, cabbage, and pumpkin. You should normally eat as much green leafy vegetables as you can unless you are on blood thinners like Warfarin for your heart. If that is the case, please consult your healthcare provider before any changes in your diet, including taking supplements. Otherwise, eat all the kale you want. Vitamin K is very important so you don't spring a leak! Please keep in mind that the RDA for Vitamin K is between 60-80 mcg.[53]

MINERALS

Go mining for minerals with your vegan diet! We often hear about the importance of maintaining the electrolyte balance. Well, that's just what the minerals are--electrolytes. Try to get these minerals naturally from food, and if you sweat a whole bunch, feel free to drink a Gatorade. Don't overdo it with electrolyte beverages, though, or you'll be swilling extra sugar water for nothing!

Calcium is important for strong bones. In America we have been duped into believing we need to get our calcium from dairy, but let's think about this. The reason milk has calcium in it is because cows eat plants. Why not just leave the animals alone and eat the plants directly? You can get 20% of your RDA from a cup of kale, collard greens, or turnip greens. Or, you can get it from fortified foods like my Silk Chocolate Soy Milk (45% RDA 1 8oz cup). Silk isn't giving me a dime to plug their stuff; it is just good.

Becoming Vegan makes some pretty good points about Calcium:[54]

1. The amount of calcium you need depends on the individual.
2. Adults generally need between 1,000 mg- 1,200 mg of calcium per day.
3. Sodium consumption blocks the intake of calcium. (Keep sodium under 2400 mg/day.)
4. Weight-bearing exercises keep your bones nice and strong.
5. Keep your protein intake within recommended levels, but don't overdo it.

Copper is important for hemoglobin synthesis which helps with oxygenation of the body. It also plays a hand in energy production and cardiac function. As far as foods go, kale is the super food, having 75% of the RDA in just 1 cup of kale. *Becoming Vegan* puts the RDA at just 0.9 mg/daily for both men and women.[55]

Iron is essential in the formation of red blood cells, which are responsible for transporting oxygen throughout the body. Not having enough iron will result in anemia, which really sucks, and will mess you up! The good news is vegan diets are generally equal to meat-eating diets in iron, so be not afraid, buckaroos! According to *Becoming Vegan*, the RDA for men is 14.4mg of iron daily, with women needing between 14.4-32.4 mg daily.[56] Squash and pumpkin seeds have the most iron of any plant-based material, with 83% of the RDA in just a 1 oz. serving. Though they pack a lower percentage of iron, cashews, peanuts, and almonds are also an okay source, giving us 34% of RDA of iron. If you think you are iron-deficient, then get your levels checked out!

Magnesium is important in the prevention of Cardiac Arrhythmias. As an RN, I can't tell you how many times I have hung a bag of IV Mag on a patient who had cardiac issues. My judgment: don't become deficient! Vegan sources include leafy green vegetables, nuts, seeds, beans, avocados, dried fruit, and dark chocolate. Per *Becoming Vegan*, men need about 400-420 mg/daily, women a little less at 310-320 mg/daily.[57]

Potassium is an important mineral for keeping a good electrolyte balance in the body. It is also very important in the regulation of nerve impulses, and in keeping the heart functioning properly. You may be interested in knowing that the infamous "lethal injection" is made up of Potassium Chloride. Not enough potassium and the heart doesn't beat right. Too much and it doesn't beat at all! Luckily, it would be very difficult to eat enough bananas to have that effect. One cup of white beans, spinach, and potatoes each has about 15% of the RDA of Potassium, and one banana has about 10% of your RDA of potassium in it. *Becoming Vegan* states that the RDA of potassium is between 2-3.5 mg for both men and women.[58]

Sodium is an important electrolyte for nerve and muscle contractions. It is essential for fluid and acid-base balance. Most of the sodium you need is already in your daily diet, and if you lose a lot of fluid, either through sweat, vomit, or urine, try to replace this electrolyte with a Gatorade or you'll be headed to the hospital for an IV. Chances are, no matter what your diet, you get enough sodium already, so avoid dousing your food with it. If you are in the hospital, we will know what your sodium level is with a blood test.

Zinc is involved in the formation of proteins, skeletal muscle formation, neurologic functions, and wound healing. The reason lozenges contain zinc is that zinc allegedly increases resistance to infections. In foods, wheat germ has the most zinc for us vegans per oz. at 111% of RDA. Pumpkin seeds have 69% per oz., which isn't too bad. There are also a lot of zinc-fortified foods out there, and so being deficient shouldn't be at the top of your worry list. Per *Becoming Vegan*, while the RDA of zinc is 11 mg for men, and about 8 mg for women, there is no single, specific, and accurate indicator of zinc's status.[59]

I highly recommend these books for more information:

- *Becoming Vegan: The Complete Guide to Adopting a Healthy Plant-Based Diet*, Brenda Davis, RD & Vesanto Melina, MS, RD, Book Publishing Company, 2000
- This is a great book and resource guide for vitamins, specific vegan nutrition questions, and general vegan health resource. I used this book while I was in vegan culinary school. Great stuff!
- Patricia Deuster, PHD, Et al *The US Navy Seal Guide to Fitness and Nutrition*, Skyhorse Publishing, Inc., 2007.
- This is where I got the calorie charts and some of the vitamin/mineral charts._*The US Navy Seal Guide to Fitness and Nutrition* is a great resource for anyone trying to get in shape.

Matt Ruscigno

Vegan Nutritionist, MPH, RD,
Chief Nutrition Officer at Nutrinic, a plant-based nutrition
center focused on cardiovascular disease prevention.
Singer in punk band H2O

How long have you been vegan?

I have been vegan since June of 1996. The day of my high school graduation. As of time of writing that's over 21 years!

Why did you go vegan and why are you still vegan?

I went vegan out of ethical concerns for animals. I had toyed with vegetarianism as a kid, twice, because I didn't want to eat animals, but I didn't know any vegetarians and didn't have the support I needed. When I learned about veganism at age 17 and met vegans, I was all the way in. It made perfect sense to me and aligned with who I wanted to be.

Not long after I decided to study nutrition in college. Not because I thought veganism was the best diet, but because I wanted to learn all I could in order to help people who also wanted to stop eating animal foods, no matter their reason. And here I am two decades later working as a nutrition professional doing exactly that.

How does being vegan affect your life/influence the direction you have gone in life?

Like a lot of people who have come out of the punk music scene, everything I do is related. For example, cycling isn't just a fun hobby- it's my community and it's a way I can work to make the world a better place. I want other people to ride bikes because it's fun and exciting and because it's good for the

101

world. Veganism is the same way. It's a big part of my personal life and obviously a major component to my career. I couldn't imagine life any other way; the personal is the political.

As a Registered Dietician, how do you feel about the soy controversy? Some people are pro, some are anti, and some don't care...

The controversy around soy is overblown. The bulk of the scientific evidence points to the health benefits of eating it. Most criticisms are exaggerations of the science or completely unscientific. They are scare tactics to keep people from changing what they eat. And if you want to be vegan but not eat soy, go right ahead! It is possible, though you'd be missing out on some great soy foods. And I'll add that it's a misnomer that populations who have been eating soy for literally centuries (primarily in Asian countries) eat only fermented soy. They eat all kinds!

Any special advice for raising vegan children?

All parents should learn about childhood nutrition, not just vegans, but for the latter it is especially important. Children have different protein needs and much smaller stomachs, so they can't eat huge amounts of whole plant foods. Reed Mangels, PhD, RD is an excellent resource on this topic. I advise future and new parents to meet with an RD who is familiar with vegan diets and working with children.

As a Registered Dietitian, do you have any advice for new vegans?

Do it your own way! Ten different vegans will give you 10 different ways that you 'must' do it. The one that matters is the one that works for you. Don't get caught up in being overly restrictive. Local is great, organic is great, but those are different things than veganism. Start with where you are now and veganize your meals. Incorporate more of the plant foods you already eat and take your time trying new foods.

Also remember that the evidence points to eating more plant foods as the most beneficial diet for health, but that doesn't mean all vegan diets are automatically healthier. Eating those plant foods is what's most important for personal health, and being vegan is what's important for the animals.

Favorite restaurants?

Big question! All-time favorite might be Happy Family 3 in Monterrey Park since it has been my go to place for big get-togethers for the last 15 years. Also Thai Food Express in MacArthur Park (Los Angeles) as it's a tiny hole in the wall that serves Northern Thai food with lots of vegan options, including mock chicken. The best Tom Kai and Tom Yum I've ever had. A new favorite spot is Bo De Tinh Tam Chay in Westminster: they have an incredibly huge menu, maybe the most intimidating one I have ever read. Those hot pots!

What else are you up to?

Right now my focus in on Nutrinic, but I still do a lot of speaking and presentations at professional conferences and veg fests. Public speaking is one of my favorite things and I do everything I can to get to places I'm invited to. My social media is instagram.com/mattruscigno and twitter.com/mattruscigno

Chapter 15

Vegan Fitness

"If they tell you to eat more meat to be strong, don't buy it."

-Arnold Schwarzenegger

I WAS NOT ATHLETIC AS A KID growing up. I didn't get into playing sports and working out until I was a freshman in high school, first with track and then wrestling. I only mention this because my athletic accomplishments happened from my late teens onward, by which time I had already gone vegan. I was 150 lbs. in high school, and as a senior in high school I wrestled in the 168 or 186 lb. spot, but only weighed about 160 lbs. soaking wet. I now weigh 190 lbs. and remain in good shape, just with more muscle. There are more accomplished athletes than myself out there obviously, even more accomplished vegan athletes, but I don't think there are as many athletes with as varied a fitness resume as myself.

► Completed 2 marathons: Japan, 1998, and Philadelphia, 2002
► Completed four ½ marathons. All in Japan.
► Completed 1 year of Senshusei Course (Intensive 6 hours a day, 5 days a week training as Aikido student in Yoshinkan Honbu Dojo, Tokyo, Japan)

- ▶ Completed 1 year as assistant teacher for Senshusei Course
- ▶ Competed California challenge in 2012 – Surf, snowboard, and skateboarded all in one day --not so much of an accomplishment as it was a really fun day.
- ▶ Army PT test score- highest 299/300, only missed perfect score because of run by 10 seconds.
- ▶ Member of First Platoon 1/508 when they won the Red Devil Challenge in 2004; (24 hours of running, shooting, and military field exercises)
- ▶ Two months kickboxing training in Thailand (1990s)
- ▶ Over 500 miles hiked on the AT (not in one day)
- ▶ Max of 5 minutes of "plank" held
- ▶ Bench Max: 270 (in 2005 while in the Army)
- ▶ Pull up Max: 20
- ▶ Push up max: 80 in 2 minutes
- ▶ Sit-up Max: 86 in 2 minutes

My goal has always been to be the best ME possible, not to be better than others. Before we begin, the most important advice I can give you about exercise is to work out SAFE and SMART! You want to train harder every day, but you also don't want to get hurt, so use the most important muscle in your body every day-your brain. When in doubt FLEX YOUR HEAD!

Running a Marathon

So you want to run a marathon? If I did it, then literally almost everyone can. Running a marathon used to seem like a lofty, hard to achieve goal, left only to the professionals. These days running a marathon is within almost everyone's reach. I say almost everyone because there are some people who shouldn't consider something like this. First, you should always check with your doctor before starting a new workout plan. If you are extremely overweight, or you have a heart problem, then you should consider a different goal. Use some common sense: don't try to run a marathon if you can't do a 5K. Also, there is a considerable amount of training that you should do before you run a marathon. There are many people who won't have the time to put into training for this.

With that in mind, here are my tips for running a marathon:

1. Train in good shoes, and change your shoes every 3 months if you are running a lot. They wear out sooner than you would think, and if you don't change them you can get shin splints.

2. Don't run every day. You need to give your muscles a chance to repair.

3. Vary your running regimen. Have some days be long run days, and other days do sprint training.

4. It will take between 3 to 6 months of training to build up to being able to run the entire marathon distance, depending on age and what kind of shape you are in when you start training.

5. Preparing for a marathon is as much about training your mind as it is for training your body. When people talk about hitting a wall after running a great distance, they aren't making it up! Understand that now, and you will be ready for that wall on mile 18.

6. Two weeks before the race, you should have worked your way up to being able to run a full 26.2 miles. That way, on game day your body won't be surprised by the sheer amount of suck that it is going through. Make sure you don't train hard in the week leading up to the big event, and take it especially easy the day before, with only a nice stretch.

7. Eat right. You need to eat at least your regular amount of food, because you will be burning a lot of calories while you are marathoning. I think it is best to run with food in your stomach, but not immediately after eating. Give your food about an hour to digest, or you will be seeing your

meal again and you won't want to post that photo on Facebook. For your pre-marathon meal, I recommend a bagel 1 hour or so before you run, but do what works for you.

8. Hydrate!! I can't emphasize this enough. H20 (water, not the influential hardcore band) is a basic building block in all life on this planet. More than half of the planet is covered in it, and you are about 70% water. (SGT VEGAN NOTE: In my case I am only 50% water. The rest is a combination of coffee and testosterone.) Anyway, water is important for all bodily functions, from being able to move waste through the body to being able to perform in a sporting competition, to thinking. Not drinking enough water can also cause hypovolemia, meaning not enough volume, which translates to low blood pressure- which can cause you to pass out. Unless you have Congestive Heart Failure or another medical condition that specifically limits your water consumption, please drink at least 64oz. of water a day (2 liters, or the usual 8 x8 cups) to optimize hydration. If you are working out, or it is hot out and you are sweating, you might need to go to 3 liters. In training – for Aikido, or in the Army- I was often drinking 3 liters a day or more. Your urine will tell you how much you need to drink. If you are peeing clear, keep up the good work. You are drinking enough water. Peeing a lemon-lime Gatorade-looking yellow? You need to drink more water, just don't go overboard. There have been cases where people have died from drinking too much water at once. Drinking too much water can lead to "hyponatremia," a condition when all of your electrolytes have been flushed out of the body. So while hydration is good, too much of a good thing is clearly not a good thing. Per the American Chemistry Society on a YouTube video, drinking 6 L of water at once will kill you. So think 2-3 L, and spread that out among the whole day, and if you are hiking, lifting, or running, or in a

hot environment, keep constantly sipping, with an electrolyte beverage every 2 hours if possible.

9. Stretch and warm up before you run. You probably already know this but I'm telling you anyway! Stretching pre and post run will not only improve your performance but also limit the chances of getting hurt, and aid in recovery time afterwards. I know that means you are going to be running a bit before you run the marathon, but trust me, it will pay off.

Go PRIMAL with Fitness

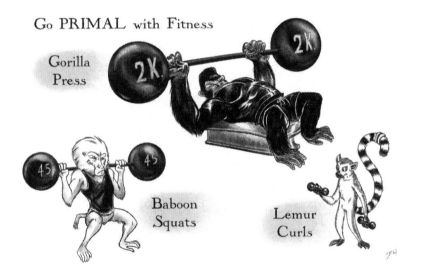

Gorilla Press

Baboon Squats

Lemur Curls

Vegan Weightlifting

I've gained 30 lbs. of muscles since I went vegan and started lifting weights. While this might have been surprising years ago, the stereotype that vegans are skinny and frail has become a thing of the past. There are many accomplished vegan bodybuilders, such as Robert Cheeke, or Korin Sutton, and I suggest you read their books as well. The following weightlifting advice might be too basic for some and too complex for others. Please check with your doctor before starting any new workout plan, always stretch and warm-up before working out, and try to have fun when you go workout. Gym time is "me time."

When you first start lifting weights, I suggest that you do a circuit 3 times a week. I would suggest Monday, Wednesday, and Friday. In this plan, you target all the major muscle groups in the body each time you lift. Here is the suggested workout:

1. **Chest**: 1. Barbell Bench Press. Warm up with a weight you can comfortably lift ten times. Then do 3 sets of a weight that you can only lift 6-8 times. Lastly, do a set of the weight you can do 10 times, and do it as many times as you can, as a burn-out set. You can change this up by using dumbbells instead of barbells. Lift the weight with control (don't bounce the bar off your chest), and go down to at least 90 degrees, where your arms make an "L" shape. 2. Incline and decline bench press: do the same thing as with barbell bench on flat bench.

2. **Shoulders** and back: Military Press, 4 sets, including 1 warm up. Use dumbbells, and go light at first. Then do 3 sets of pull-ups, feeling free to use the pull-up machine to make it easier if you need it. Seated row: 4 sets, including warm up. Make sure you keep your back straight, and always lift with good form.

3. **Legs**: Squat. With or without weight. Legs should be shoulder width apart, toes pointing straight out, squat down keeping your back straight and try to go down to a 90-degree angle. Squat leg press. 4 times, and do a set of calf raises after each set of leg press, making sure that the guard is up so you don't drop the weight on yourself. Leg Extension. 4 times.

4. **Arms**: Biceps 1. Standing curls with dumbbells. 4 sets, alternating each arm, 10 reps each arm. 2. Then do 21s — using a curl bar, do 7 reps halfway up, 7 reps halfway to the top, and 7 reps bottom to top. Repeat for 3 sets. Triceps extension with rope: Stand with rope about 5 inches from

you, and elbows close to your body and facing down. With control, bring rope down in front of you and flare your arms out as you do. Do 4 sets, and if you have never done this exercise before there are a lot of great videos on YouTube that you can watch.

SGT Vegan's Training Tips:

1. The triceps muscle makes up most of your upper arm, so if you want bigger arms, you have to concentrate on your triceps. Once you have the swing of the above workout, add in skull crushers (GOOGLE IT) to make it count!

2. Make sure you get adequate rest and fluids. You are going to need at least 2 days for the muscle to heal in between workouts.

3. Eat 20 grams of quality protein within one hour after your workout. This is the golden hour, when your muscles need it most.

4. Raise the weight by 5 lbs. after the weight that you are doing gets easy enough that you could do it for 10 reps.

5. Listen to some music that cranks up your adrenaline. Lift with a partner who motivates you to lift harder. Have fun; it will make you want to come back for more.

6. Try not to have competing goals fitness goals. You can train for a marathon and you can lift weights, but realize that running will naturally slim your body down. If you are trying to bulk up, running far distances will be counter-productive, and vice-versa.

7. Make sure you warm up your muscles before you lift heavy. You can do this with a little cardio on the treadmill, and by lifting the bar with good form to warm up before you start killing it.

8. Always lift with good form, and don't cheat!

9. Write down how much you are lifting at the start of your program, and keep track your progress every workout. You won't know how far you've come if you forget where you started!

LEVEL UP:

The split schedule! Once you have been lifting for a couple of months and you want to get serious about it, it's time to do a split schedule. This means that you can lift almost every day, because you only lift with one or 2 body parts at a time and can rest the other body parts while lifting with another part.

1. Chest and Triceps
2. Back and Biceps
3. Shoulders/legs
4. Repeat

Sooner or later you will start to plateau. When you do, you need to change up your exercises and keep your muscles from getting comfortable.

Weight Lifting Supplements

Creatine. This is a substance that the body makes naturally in small quantities, and that meat eaters get when they eat the flesh of animals. Vegans can get a synthetic supplement version made in a lab without animal involvement. The reasoning behind using creatine is that it helps get more water into the muscles, which then makes the muscles repair themselves quicker, allowing you to work out longer and make more gains. I feel like creatine might have helped when I was lifting a lot. The downside was it made me look and feel a little "puffy" and bloated with all of the extra water in my muscles. If you decide to take creatine, make sure you drink enough water. Since people need to be drinking at least 2 liters a day normally, try to drink 3 liters daily so you can flush out your kidneys. The people who experienced adverse reactions (some very serious) all had complications from problems with their kidneys, which could have been avoided with adequate hydration. Use with caution!!

Protein Powders. The cheaper protein powders aren't very delicious. I occasionally take the Vega protein, and in a properly-made shake (frozen banana, Silk soy milk) it isn't bad. Everyone you talk to has a different opinion about protein intake. Generally, most bodybuilders will say take a gram per kilogram of body weight. As stated before, it is important to get about 20 grams of protein right after working out, either in a shake or protein bar form. Some bodybuilders also drink a shake before going to sleep with the idea that your body has nutrition and it is not starved overnight. I see where they are coming from, but I like a couple of hours with nothing in my stomach before I go to sleep myself.

The Vegan Bodybuilder Interviews

Robert Cheeke

Author, Athlete, Entrepreneur
Founder/President of Vegan Bodybuilding & Fitness
<u>*www.veganbodybuilding.com*</u>

How long have you been vegan?

I have been vegan since December 8, 1995.

Why did you go vegan and why are you still vegan?

I grew up on a farm in the agricultural town of Corvallis, Oregon, and developed an appreciation for farm animals similar to the respect and appreciation someone might have for a dog or a cat. Given this perspective and my closeness to animals – raising them as pets – through my involvement in 4-H, it seemed fitting to stop eating my animal friends. In the mid 90's, as a teenager, I no longer wanted to contribute to animal cruelty and suffering and decided to go vegan. When I became vegan in 1995, I was 15 years old and weighed 120 pounds. By 2003, I was up to 195 pounds and was a competitive bodybuilder.

The reasons I am vegan today, more than twenty years after I adopted this lifestyle, are the same reasons that inspired me to go vegan in the first place. My desire is to reduce animal suffering and cruelty, and to save animal lives. I do that through living a vegan lifestyle and by spreading the message from writing books, touring, speaking, and writing for numerous media publications.

How has being vegan changed your life?

I've often said that the decision I made on that December day back in 1995 to become vegan changed my life forever. I'd like to think that becoming vegan has made me a more compassionate person in all aspects of life. I feel like living a cruelty-free lifestyle strengthens my desire to help human and non-human animals alike. Living this way has enabled me to stand out in the athletic world, succeed as an author, and has given me a platform to influence many people. My goal is to be healthy, happy, and fit, and to lead by positive example.

Tell me about something cool you've done.

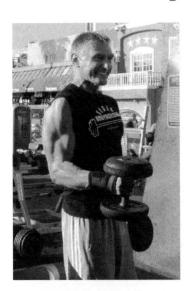

Robert Cheeke

Some of the things I am proudest of were accomplished in my mid-twenties. In 2005 I filmed a documentary titled *Vegan Fitness – Built Naturally*, and I created The Vegan Vacation (2006-2008), and The Vegan Holiday Festival (2006-2007). Additionally, I released my first book, *Vegan Bodybuilding & Fitness*, in 2010, and my second book, *Shred It!* which I am really enthusiastic about, in 2014. Most recently, the coolest thing I've done for my personal enrichment is tour with my new book in Australia, the Caribbean, eastern and western Canada, and across the USA. It has truly been a rewarding journey.

Advice for new vegans?

My advice to those who are new to the vegan lifestyle is to find deep meaning in your reasons for being vegan. The more meaningful your reasons for living a compassionate, cruelty-free life, the more likely you will keep this lifestyle for the long term. Focus on the issues that matter most to you, that touch your heart, and work hard to be a compassionate person to all living beings. Nutritionally, focus on nutrient-dense whole foods, such as fruits, vegetables, nuts, grains, seeds, and legumes. Read books, become part of online vegan communities, and network with others. Find enjoyable forms of exercise and train hard, eat well, smile often, and lift others up.

Favorite cuisines?

My favorite meal is a simple one. I really enjoy brown rice, pinto and black beans, avocado, lettuce, tomato, and salsa. I also greatly enjoy Ethiopian, Indian, Thai, and Japanese cuisine in addition to Mexican cuisine, which is the foundation of my favorite meal.

Thank you for taking the opportunity to interview me. Readers can find me on Twitter at @RobertCheeke, on Facebook under Robert Cheeke, and on www.veganbodybuilding.com.

KORIN SUTTON

Personal Trainer, Pro Bodybuilder

How long have you been vegan?

I have been vegan since 2012.

Why did you go vegan and why are you still vegan?

I am vegan because I feel that there is no difference between all living beings on this planet. We should all share this planet as one and try to cause the least amount of violence and damage

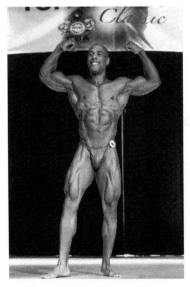

Korin Sutton

to it if we want this planet to survive for years to come. This planet is a living organism and we should take care of it, including the other living species who cohabitate with us. During this day and age, animals are being mistreated, raped, tortured, enslaved, and killed everyday for human consumption and entertainment. I believe this is wrong on all levels.

With today's food technology we do not have to live off of other animals for our simple pleasures. We have animal food replacements or "veganized" foods which are cruelty free, non-GMO, and a lot healthier for human consumption. By being vegan, people live longer, healthier lives, and can rest easy knowing that they are not participating in any hatred or cruelty toward other living species. Eating a plant-based diet has so many health benefits, and knowing this is why I'm vegan and in the health care and exercise science profession. I can teach other people how to live a healthier and cruelty- free life style not only to benefit themselves but also other living species and the environment too.

How has being vegan changed your life?

My favorite thing about being vegan is living with a clearer conscience, knowing that this is the most compassionate way to live. Being vegan to me is not just about "eating clean," but it has also made me more spiritual. I was in the military for about 8 years, 4 years active United States Marine Corps, and 4 years as an active reservist in The United States Navy. I remember that I would have minor cases of PTSD in the past which I never reported to the VA Department, just because I thought I would be considered weak for not being able to handle my own demons. Now my mind is clearer and silent because I am vegan. I'm a true believer that you are what you eat, and if you are spiritual why consume animals that have been slaughtered, raped, enslaved, and tortured. This is all negative energy that you are consuming and it shows. I noticed it myself, and I had to walk away from eating meat and supporting that cause. Now I practice and follow Buddhism which has also helped me throughout my journey.

Tell me about something cool you've done.

I've been with PlantBuilt Vegan Muscle Team for about 1 1/2 years. In 2014 PlantBuilt raised over $40,000 dollars to help promote veganism and also to donate to animal sanctuaries. Now we are trying to raise over $50,000. PlantBuilt is a non-profit organization and as a collective of athletes we live, train, compete, and educate communities, showing the successful lifestyle of compassionate veganism. Find me on YouTube under Vegan Live Fit.

Chapter 16

"Dieting" Cliff Notes

"The solution to losing weight is a whole-food, plant-based diet, coupled with a reasonable amount of exercise. It is a long-term lifestyle change, rather than a quick-fix fad, and it can provide sustained weight loss while minimizing risk of chronic disease."[60]

- Dr. Colin T. Campbell, The China Study

I BELIEVE IF YOU HAVE THOROUGHLY read this book, this chapter won't be necessary, but I don't live in a fantasy world. Let's face it; we Americans can be a little lazy sometimes, and life is fast-paced. As long as you are getting out to exercise and eat vegan, I promise not to call you out on your reading habits. Deal?

Eating healthy should not be thought of as a temporary habit; rather, it should be a permanent change in the way you live. Except for this chapter, when I use the word "diet," I am using the term in the medical way to describe a system of eating, NOT to mean a reduction of calories. Short-term reductions in calories, especially starvation diets, create an unhealthy yo-yo effect in your body. Extremes are often negative, whether they are changes in the climate or in your body. To eat a "vegan diet," on the other hand, should be thought of as a return to what you should have been doing all along. No worries, this chapter is here to help!

The key to maintaining a healthy weight is calories: calories in vs calories out. As long as you are expending more calories than you take in, you will not gain weight. If you expend more than you take in, you will lose weight. It is imperative you do this in a measured, slow way. Most people put on weight over time, and not in a matter of weeks, so move slowly with a plan and conviction and you will lose weight. Going about this as a mad dash will usually result in failure and grumpiness, with no overall weight loss, and possible health risks.

Calories are not the enemy. Calories fuel your life. We need carbohydrates, proteins, and fats in our daily life. Since I already went into the nutritional breakdown in previous chapters, I won't repeat that part here. However, I will say this: avoid empty calories! An empty calorie does not provide any necessary macro or micro nutrients or fiber, but instead just turns to body fat. Examples: Cookies, cake, candy, chips, French fries, etc. Try to limit them, for they are bad food choices. If you need to eat dessert, turn to fruit.

The following is a collection of tips about losing weight and getting in shape listed in easily digestible bullet points. You are welcome.

1. Drink at least 2 liters of water a day. Remember the 8 cups of water a day? That comes out to 2L-- 8x8 oz.= 64 oz., or 2 liters. That is the recommended amount of water that you should be drinking a day to sustain your body functions. (SGT VEGAN NOTE: Drink that or maybe a little more than that, but remember NOT to overdo it on water, especially in one sitting! People have died from drinking too much water at once!)

2. Don't drink your calories! Soda, juice, beer, whatever it is, if it contains calories you shouldn't be drinking it. If you drink coffee, drink it black. A smoothie is okay if you are doing it as a meal replacement as long as you are getting all

of your daily RDA of vitamins, minerals, and enough protein. Drinking a smoothie when you are thirsty is bad. In other words, if you are thirsty, reach for water.

3. Find out how many calories you need to sustain your current body weight; the equation is found in the previous chapter (REE). Most people are eating way more than they should, and unspent calories, especially empty calories, means weight gain. To find out what your average caloric intake is, and to see what your eating trends are, keep a food diary for one week. Count up your daily caloric intake, and see where you are. If you are right around where your daily intake should be, good work! If you are way over your calorie limit, consider making better food choices, and limiting portion sizes of junk foods. Most importantly, don't starve yourself! Long-term goals will only be met with slow, steady, measured progress. Starving yourself will hurt you in the long run, and impede long-term success. Think of getting to your target healthy weight as a marathon and not a sprint.

4. Fruits and vegetables are good! Unless you are on blood thinners or are allergic to any fruits and vegetables, consider this your invitation to eat as many of them as you want, within reason. I mean within reason because fruits and vegetables are great ways to get fiber, and they contain very little calories as is, but loaded down with dressing or sautéed in oil, they are a fatty mess. So when you eat salad, be careful about the salad dressing, which often adds additional fat and calories. When cooking vegetables, aim to steam, sauté in water, or grill them. Frying, especially with oil, adds empty calories. Avoid fried foods like the plague. Treat yourself right; don't abuse your body by eating fried garbage.

5. The timing of your meals is crucial. No matter when you wake up, breakfast is still the most important meal of the day. Remember breakfast means "break the fast." Don't

skip breakfast and think you are going to save the calories in a bank and eat them up later. Your body doesn't work that way. Spread your meals out through the day with the traditional breakfast, lunch, and dinner format, with healthy snacks in between lunch and dinner: a piece of fruit or a handful of nuts. Eat slowly, chewing each bite of your food, and take sips of water between bites. Doing this will give your brain the time it needs to realize you are full.

6. The importance of exercise to weight loss is not to be understated. Please consult your physician to determine that you are healthy enough to start any exercise program. Walking is a great first step (pun intended) towards fitness, as it generally has a lower impact on the joints than any other cardiovascular workout, with the exception of swimming. Swimming is great exercise, has even lower impact on your joints than walking, but requires access to a pool, lake, ocean, or other body of water, and of course the ability to swim. Floating/bobbing around a pool while doing your best impression of an ice cube in a cup of lemonade is not exercise. Walking requires simply having two legs that are in working order, and an operational heart/respiratory system. When you first start on the path to fitness, you should walk 30 minutes 3x a week as your exercise, with the goal of eventually walking an hour every day. I also recommend a pedometer, be it a "Fit Bit" or an app on your phone. This will let you keep track of the distance that you go every day so you can monitor your progress. Once you are comfortable with walking as an exercise, and your doctor has cleared you to start exercising more vigorously, move on to a weight- bearing exercise regime as described in the Chapter "Vegan Fitness."

Chapter 17

A Word on FAD Diets

BY NOW I HOPE YOU HAVE LEARNED that balance is key when it comes to successful nutrition in a vegan diet. In previous chapters we have learned the proper amount of energy (calories), macros (carbs, protein, fat), and micros (vitamins and minerals) the body needs to thrive on a vegan diet. I feel the following fad diets are not as effective as living a healthy vegan life because of their inability to optimize the healthy balance of nutrition necessary from eating a variety of fruits and vegetables, and whole grains.

Gluten-Free

The Good:
   Brought awareness to the plight of those with celiac disease.

The Bad:
   For people who aren't celiac, Gluten-Free is a waste of time and money.

The first of the fad diets is gluten-free. Gluten is a part of the wheat plant that gives it protein. It is used in baking bread to make the dough stronger, and it gives bread an edge in making it a nutrient-rich food if it is made right. This diet came to prominence with acknowledging that some people are allergic to gluten. According to the National Foundation for Celiac Awareness, about one in a hundred people is allergic to gluten and products that contain gluten – that's only 1% of the U.S. population. In the same way nuts are healthy and good for you unless you have a nut allergy, products with gluten are fine unless you have celiac disease. There is no reason to buy gluten-free if you don't have problems consuming wheat.[61] (SGT VEGAN NOTE: It would be like carrying an M-16 when you really want an M-4. I'm looking at you, Marines!). Gluten-free also tends to be more expensive because manufacturers are taking advantage of clueless shoppers, and the products are rarely as good as their wheat-containing original counterparts. Take SGT Vegan's advice: If you think you are allergic to anything, then get tested. Knowledge is power! If you aren't celiac, then go ahead, drop a sensible portion of whole grain pasta on your plate and don't give it a second thought. And a word to manufacturers: Please don't be lazy and lump vegan and gluten-free together. We get why you are putting the two things together, to make something for all of us "fussy eaters," but if I am eating a vegan cookie, I'm okay with it having wheat in it. Making a one-size- fits- all product for every "fussy eater" is a sure-fire way to ensure you make something that sucks for everyone. Instead of eating your "wheat free, sugar free, fat free, taste free cookie" I'll just have a banana instead.

The take away:

If you think you might be gluten-sensitive, by all means, get tested to see if you are allergic. Otherwise, eating Gluten-Free might be a waste of your money.

Paleo Diet

The Good:

This diet is all about cutting out chemicals and modern day BS from our diets.

The Bad:

The cavemen's life expectancy was short. Dying young is only cool if you are a punk-rocker in 1979.

So the Paleo diet (short for Paleolithic or the caveman era) was dreamed up as a way to get away from the modern Standard-American Diet. Its creators were correct that extra sweeteners and chemicals are detrimental to health, and they were also correct people should be eating more vegetables. Where they went wrong was their assumption our cavemen ancestors were healthy to begin with. Spoiler alert: they weren't. The average life expectancy of a caveman was 35 years old. Cavemen ate a diet high in meat because they didn't have a lot of other options. As we have seen earlier in this book, eating meat can lead to a plethora of medical issues (cardiac and others). Of course, if you were a caveman who had to worry about being eaten by a saber tooth tiger, you probably didn't care about the modern day cardiac killers because you wouldn't live long enough for them to catch up with you. In a way, this meat-heavy diet is something of a re-packaged Atkins Diet for the cross-fit generation.

The take away:

The paleo diet is right to avoid eating processed junk, but don't be a caveman! Eat like an enlightened being from our modern times with the best scientific advice at your fingertips. In other words, eat vegan food, but avoid processed junk. Remember, cavemen didn't know anything about science or nutrition; they worshiped the stars and were afraid of fire. Do you really want to take nutritional advice from them?

Atkins Diet

The Good:

Not much.

The Bad:

Heavy in animal proteins, which are bad for the kidneys; high in animal fat which causes heart attacks.

The Atkins diet is similar to the Paleo Diet in that it is heavy in proteins and lets you eat all the meat you want. You cut out carbs, so that limits calories, which is why some people experience weight loss. Where it differs from the Paleo Diet is that the Atkins diet doesn't tend to recommend all of the vegetables Paleo encourages you to eat. While a lot of the Paleo people tend to be the Cross-Fit types who are healthier than the average American, people on the Atkins diet tend to be obese and are just trying to lose weight. As mentioned earlier, Atkins himself might have died due to complications related to following his own advice.[62]

The Take Away:

Stay away from the processed crap and the Atkins Diet.

Fruitarian

The Good:

High in Vitamin C

The Bad:

Do you really want to eat 20 bananas a day?

I've met some people living on a fruitarian diet. Being a fruitarian is similar to the raw vegan diet except you are only eating fruit. It is extremely difficult to eat a balanced diet without vegetables and whole grains. This diet is hard to stick with and can make you quite sick. Just ask Steve Jobs, lifelong Fruitarian. Unfortunately, you can't, because he is dead, and his diet might have contributed to his death. As Ashton Kutcher found out the hard way when he got sick after eating only fruit for a month in an attempt to prepare for his role as Steve Jobs, this diet is not a great idea.[63]

The Take Away:

Please continue to eat fruit daily, but make sure you eat whole grains and vegetables as well.

Raw Vegan

The Good:
Well, it has vegan in the title.

The Bad:
No fire!

Proponents of a raw vegan diet argue that vegetables lose their nutrients when they are cooked. While some vegetables do lose their nutrients when cooked it is also true that some vegetables need to be cooked in order to unlock their full nutrient potential. Unlike rapper Ol' Dirty Bastard, who in the second track of his 1995 solo album "Return to the 36 Chambers" proclaimed "Oh Baby I like it Raw," I think most of us actually like "it" cooked -- our veggies that is. Yes, broccoli loses about 10% of its Vitamin C when you steam it, but you could just make up for that by eating another piece of broccoli to make up the difference, unless you also "Like it Raw."[64] According to *How Not To Die*, vegetables such as carrots, celery, and green beans actually become better for you when being cooked, needing heat to unlock their antioxidant potential no matter what the method you use.[65] The bottom line: eat lots of veggies. Eat them raw, cooked, upside and down, whatever way you want; just eat lots of vegetables.

The Take Away:
Generally, as long as you aren't deep frying, or boiling the heck out of your vegetables, I think you are good to go to use a variety of cooking (or lack of cooking) methods to prepare nature's bounty for yourself and your family. (SGT Vegan Alert: Deep frying foods has been linked to cancer,[66] so keep your consumption of fried foods to a minimum.)

Part 3

VEGAN DELICIOUS

Chapter 18

American Vegan Food

OF COURSE THERE IS NO WAY I could write a book about vegan food and not include some recipes. The difference between my book and other vegan cookbooks is I actually use these recipes, and you don't have to travel to East Jibip to get the ingredients. I agree that variety is the spice of life, but being vegan doesn't mean you have to travel to Mars for lunch. Here is my collection of vegan recipes, the secret weapon to becoming *VEGAN STRONG*.

In addition to these recipes, I encourage you to start trying out all of the great new vegan products out there designed to make your life as a vegan easier. To be vegan, it is often as easy as substituting vegan products for their animal counterparts. Take dinner for example; you normally start with a salad. Most salad dressings can be found in an animal-free variety, and you can even find vegan Bacon Bits (SGT VEGAN NOTE: Always read the ingredient list carefully, and don't get caught with them during an Army locker inspection).

Moving on to the main course, let's say it's pasta night. Most store-bought spaghetti noodles are vegan by default, so make sure you have a vegan sauce, and you are well on your way to a delicious vegan meal. I wouldn't stop there though. Before you add the sauce, first sauté an onion, some garlic, and vegan Italian sausages by Tofurkey, or meatballs by Gardein. When you add the sauce it will have a much more flavorful taste, and then you are in veggie paradise! I think broccoli pairs well with this, so add some steamed broccoli or lightly sautéed broccoli. Broccoli is a giant in both taste and nutrition. Eat it as much as possible, but don't go overboard because it might give you some gas.

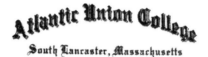

South Lancaster, Massachusetts

We hereby certify that

William F. Muir

has satisfactorily completed the curriculum in

Vegetarian/Vegan Culinary Arts

and is awarded this certificate

this eleventh day of May, 2008

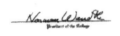 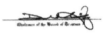

Certified Vegan Chef

PROTEINS

The Fine Art of Tofu
Scrambled, Baked, and Fried

If you have never bought tofu before, you might be a little confused when you see it in your supermarket. There are many brands, and it comes in different levels of firmness. What is the difference between brands? Usually a couple of dollars, so please find a brand you like. Many people say go for a brand that doesn't use GMOs. As for the firmness, it depends on what you want to do with it. If you are making tofu pudding, go for silken tofu. If you are making tofu scramble, baked, or fried tofu, go extra-firm. The firmness refers to the water content; the firmer the tofu, the less water it will contain.

♥ *Tofu Scramble* ♥

Do you miss eating scrambled eggs in the morning? Well, this is not exactly the same thing, but it is delicious. Served the same way you would serve any scramble, it goes great with toast, hash brown, veggie sausage, pancakes, or any other deliciousness. Store the unused portion in the refrigerator to be used later in the same breakfast fashion, or on top of salads in place of feta, or in a wrap with Vegenaise, or in potato salad in place of egg. This recipe will make about 3 servings.

You will need:
- ▶ 1 Pack of extra firm tofu
- ▶ 1 cup of broccoli or half an onion in rough- chop form. The broccoli will have more nutritional value to it, but not everyone is a fan, and the onion is more traditional.

- ► 2 tablespoons of McKay's Vegan Chicken Seasoning (available on Amazon, or at most Seventh Day Adventist Grocery Stores) or make your own-
- ► "fakey chicken seasoning"
- ► 1tsp garlic powder, 1 tsp onion powder, 1 tsp oregano (could also use 1 T Italian herbs blend instead), with a small pinch of turmeric – gives it a nice yellow color, also good for your immune system, 1 T nutritional yeast flakes, and salt to taste

Steps:

1. In a fry pan, add a small amount of olive oil or cooking spray. On medium heat, add the chopped broccoli or onion. Allow the broccoli or onion to cook until it starts to turn slightly brown (called caramelized).
2. Thoroughly drain all water from the tofu, then add it to the pan, crumbling it as you go.
3. Mix the broccoli or onion and tofu crumbles.
4. Add the seasoning, and stir. If the tofu scramble is too dry, add 1 teaspoon of warm water.

LEVEL UP:

- ► Option 1: Fold in one diced Tofurkey Italian sausage link before adding the tofu. Tofu scramble already has enough protein, so we are just adding the link for its delicious flavor.
- ► Option 2: Instead of broccoli or onions use red and yellow peppers for color contrast. This makes for a great photo to put on Instagram or FB.
- ► Option 3: Tofu Mc Muffin: Fold in Daiya Cheese at the end of cooking, allowing cheese to melt. Put cheese-infused tofu scramble on an English muffin along with a Tofurkey vegan Ham slice. Ensure the muffin is toasted until golden brown and slathered with Earth Balance buttery spread.

♥ *Herb Crusted Tofu* ♥

This method will work with tofu, seitan, eggplant, and pretty much anything as well. You could batter and fry a tire and it would taste great, just little chewy (just kidding, don't do that).

What you will need:

- ► 1 Box of Panko (Japanese Bread Crumbs)
- ► 2 T Italian Seasonings Blend (Oregano, Thyme, basil, garlic, etc.)
- ► 1 cup Soy milk (plain) or water
- ► 1 package of extra firm tofu
- ► 3 separate containers
- ► Salt and pepper to taste
- ► 1 cup All Purpose Flour (gluten free people- please use whatever kind of flour you are substituting for wheat flour

Steps:

1. Lay out your 3 containers. Place flour in the first container.
2. Place water or soy milk in the second container
3. Place 1 cup of Panko and 2 T of seasonings in the third container.
4. Now you are ready to dip. Take your medium-sized piece of tofu -- not too thin for it will fall apart, not too thick because it won't cook, and dip it first in the flour, then the water, then the panko.
5. After you are finished coating all of your pieces, place 2 T of oil in a pan (or use cooking spray) and place over a medium heat. When the oil starts to get hot, add the battered pieces, but make sure not to crowd them in the pan. After a couple of minutes flip them to make sure they get browned on both sides, and take out of pan.
6. Sprinkle some Sea Salt on the pieces, and serve with your favorite sauce.

♥ *Baked Tofu* ♥

Yes, you can even bake tofu. This is a slower, low fat option, and will result in crispy tofu pieces. There are 2 basic ways I would perform this method, either coating the pieces with panko (breadcrumbs), or dipping them in BBQ sauce and baking them.

Panko Shake-N-Bake method

1. Coat the pieces in the same manner as if you were going to fry them, but leave out the flour.
2. Spray baking sheet with fat free cooking spray or coat with olive oil.
3. Lay the pieces out evenly on the sheet.
4. Place in oven, heated to 350 degrees for 45 minutes or until the tofu browns.
5. Top with pinch of sea salt, serve with favorite sauce. Pairs well with couscous/quinoa and a vegetable like steamed broccoli or asparagus spears.

♥ *BBQ Tofu* ♥

1. Spray baking sheet with cooking/baking spray.
2. Slather the well-cut tofu pieces with BBQ sauce and arrange in an organized method on the baking tray.
3. Bake at 350 degrees for 45 minutes or when the tofu starts to get dry. Feel free to add extra BBQ sauce after cooking as you see fit.

♥ *SGT Vegan's Kickass Seitan* ♥

Seitan reigns forever, as long as you aren't on a gluten-free diet. Unless you are gluten intolerant or have Celiac's disease, seitan is a great source of protein, a super affordable alternative to commercially-made meat substitutes, and very delicious. These recipes produce a product which is very similar to meat in taste and texture, without any of the cholesterol, fat, or mistreatment of animals.

Basic Recipe –

What you will need:

- ▶ 2.25 cups of vital wheat gluten flour
- ▶ 2 tablespoons of McKay's Seasoning. Alternatives: 1 vegan ramen soup flavoring packet, or 2 T fakey chicken seasoning
- ▶ 1 and 2/3 cups warm water
- ▶ 1/3 cup soy sauce
- ▶ 1 tsp rosemary
- ▶ 1 tsp thyme
- ▶ 1 tsp oregano

What you need to do:

1. Add all wet ingredients together
2. Add all dry ingredients together separately
3. Blend both together, kneading as you mix.
4. After the wet and dry are thoroughly mixed and kneaded together, set the ball of dough aside.
5. In a separate pot, bring to a boil 6 cups of liquid (1 cup of soy sauce, 5 cups of vegetable broth, your favorite seasonings as desired)
6. Place dough ball in boiling water and cook on medium heat for an hour.
7. Remove from heat and use as you would meat in any recipe. It will be good baked, fried, sautéed.

LEVEL UP:

  After preparing the dough ball in step 4, cut it into thin strips of raw dough. Fry the pieces of dough in a frying pan with olive oil until brown on both sides. Once the pieces are fried, place all together in the water mixture in step 5 above and boil for an hour.

This method makes for better seitan to use on the grill, as the frying and then boiling makes the pieces absorb water and inflate. After these pieces boil, let them cool, then place them in a bowl with BBQ sauce and stick in the fridge for 2 hours to marinate. Now you are ready to grill and enjoy!!

SGT Vegan WARNING: the above boiling time for seitan is the minimum. You can boil the seitan a little longer, but don't undercook it or you will be eating raw flour!

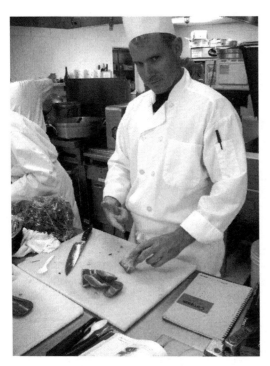

Remember to always make vegetables a big part of any meal

ENTREES

♥ *Mom's Awesome Stuffed Shells* ♥

My mom is Italian, and has veganized numerous Italian recipes for my brother and me. This is one such recipe. Get ready for pure Vegan Italian Awesomeness! This will feed a family of 4.

You will need:

- ► 1 (16 oz.) of large shells
- ► 1 jars Trader Joe's Marinara sauce (or your favorite brand)
- ► 1 large block of extra firm tofu, crumbled and drained of all liquid
- ► 2 cups of canned spinach, drained of all liquid (about 2 medium cans)
- ► 1 medium onion, peeled and chopped
- ► 3 cloves of garlic, minced
- ► cooking spray or olive oil
- ► 1/2 medium sweet red pepper, washed and diced
- ► 1 small can of mushrooms, drained and chopped
- ► 1 T Italian Seasoning, or to taste
- ► 1 tsp salt, or more to taste
- ► ¼ tsp pepper

What you do:

1. Boil the pasta shells until they are el dente (still firm, but edible) and drain them.
2. Next, in a large skillet, heat the oil or pan spray, sauté the garlic, onions, and red pepper until soft.
3. Stir. Squeeze the spinach until all of the water is out, and add to skillet. Stir.
4. Add the mushrooms. Stir.

5. Mash the tofu until it is in fine, small chunks, confirm there is no water, and add to the skillet. Stir.
6. Now sprinkle the seasoning evenly over contents and make sure it is evenly blended.
7. Add extra seasoning to taste.
8. Drain excess water from pan after cooking on medium heat for 15 minutes. Add 1 cup of spaghetti sauce. Stir. Remove from heat.
9. Get 2 large baking dishes and grease or spray pan. Add 1 cup of spaghetti sauce to the pan and distribute evenly.
10. Fill each shell with a large spoonful of mixture and line up in dish. You may need another dish to hold all of the shells.
11. When all shells are filled, place a small amount of sauce on top of each shell.
12. Cover baking pan with tin foil, and bake in an oven preheated to 350 degrees for 30-40 minutes.
13. Time will depend on your oven; start checking at 30 minutes for doneness. Remove from heat when contents are steaming. Cover with Daiya Cheese (or your favorite vegan brand) and let it melt over the shells before serving. Serve with vegan meatballs and extra sauce.

♥ *Good Shepherd's Pie* ♥

Shepherds don't eat their own flock; that's creepy. There are many variations of this recipe out there. Here is one I like.

What you will need:

- ► 13"x9" greased baking dish
- ► 1 1/2 lbs. ground (finely chopped) seitan, or other ground beef substitute
- ► 10 oz. onions, chopped
- ► 1 bag of peas, frozen (about 10 oz.)
- ► 0.5 lb. of carrots, peeled and sliced like coins
- ► 12 oz. of spaghetti sauce
- ► 2 T vegan MacKay's beef seasoning. Alternatives: Vegan ramen soup packet, or 2 T of fakey chicken seasoning
- ► salt and pepper to taste
- ► mashed potatoes for topping (see recipe)

What you do:

1. Prep seitan and fine chop
2. Sauté chopped onions in olive oil, add seitan after onions are caramelized.
3. Cook peas and carrots and drain
4. Mix all ingredients together with spaghetti sauce.
5. Spread into greased bake pan.
6. Spread cold mashed potatoes over top of mixture (see recipe below)
7. Bake in oven at 350 for 30-40 minutes. You will know the dish is ready when the mashed potatoes are lightly browned.
8. Cool, cut, and serve.
9. Can be frozen, thawed, and reheated.

♥ *BBQ Tempeh Sandwich* ♥

Tempeh, much like tofu, is not inherently delicious on its own. You have to know how to prepare it and what sauces pair well with it. The way I like to prepare tempeh is pan-fried and drowned in BBQ sauce. Here's how you do it.

What you will need:

- ► 1 bottle of your favorite BBQ sauce. Watch out for honey.
- ► 1 package of tempeh
- ► olive oil/cooking spray
- ► Vegenaise
- ► sandwich bread- preferably crusty roll or ciabatta
- ► fixings for sandwich (thick tomato and romaine lettuce for starters, maybe onion)

What your do:

1. Cut tempeh into thin strips.
2. Add olive or vegetable oil to a fry pan, or no-fat cooking spray, and simmer on medium heat
3. Add tempeh to the fry pan
4. Flip tempeh when brown.
5. When all tempeh is browned on both sides, add BBQ sauce, and thoroughly coat pieces.
6. Remove pan from heat.
7. Toast bread (ciabatta is best) and then slather with Veganaise.
8. Add BBQ Tempeh, top with lettuce and tomato, and then insert in mouth.

♥ *Mom's Vegan Chili* ♥

After having to eat chili every day for months in Afghanistan (Please see Chapter 7), you could say I have a complicated relationship with it. That being said, I have to acknowledge my Mom makes the best vegan chili in the world. If you are a chili lover you are in for a treat, and even if you aren't you will still love this. If you are a meat eater, you won't miss the meat in it. You are welcome, world.

What you will need:

- ► 1 can light red kidney beans, drained
- ► 1 can kernel corn, drained
- ► 1 can black beans, drained
- ► 1 large can of crushed tomatoes
- ► 1 medium onion, diced
- ► 1 clove of diced garlic
- ► 2 T chili powder
- ► 1 tsp cumin
- ► Diced green or red peppers, mushrooms optional

What you do:

Pan spray or olive oil sauté garlic and onions until soft in large pot. Add all other contents. Allow to simmer on medium heat for 45 minutes-1 hour. Remove from heat, serve with rice or macaroni.

LEVEL UP:

Add vegan crumbles or diced seitan, or serve with vegan cheddar cheese on top.

SIDES

♥ *Easy Mashed Potatoes* ♥

Mashed Potatoes are easy to make and here's the recipe to show you how.

You will need:

- ▶ 2 lb. potatoes (Russet or Idaho)
- ▶ 1 cup plain soymilk
- ▶ 1 T Mc Kay's Vegan Chicken Seasoning (or alternate, see previous) or more to taste
- ▶ 2 T Earth Balance Spread
- ▶ salt and pepper to taste
- ▶ 1 hand mixer

Traditional Method:

1. Peel, and cut potatoes into large cubes.
2. Boil water in big pot.
3. When water is at boil, put potato cubes in water
4. Boil until they are soft, remove from heat and pour into strainer.
5. Rinse briefly to get excess starch off potatoes.
6. Place potatoes into big bowel.
7. Add the Earth Balance spread and the seasoning
8. Using hand mixer, whip the potatoes into desired consistency, adding small amounts of soy milk as you go UNTIL you get the consistency works for you. DON'T ADD IT ALL AT ONCE!!! You want to avoid accidentally making potato soup.
9. Salt and Pepper to taste. Serve hot with extra Earth Balance.

Alternative Method:

I came up with this recently, as a way to avoid the work in making mashed potatoes. This method is slightly risky because you can get the consistency wrong. On the other hand, it is a lot less time consuming. Also, apparently eating potato skins is good for you.

What you will need:

- ▶ 4 medium sized potatoes
- ▶ 1 T McKay's Vegan Chicken Seasoning.
- ▶ salt and pepper to taste
- ▶ 1 T Earth Balance spread\
- ▶ 1 T Vegenaise or similar vegan mayo spread
- ▶ Cuisinart food processor

What you will do:

1. Thoroughly clean all potatoes, and poke holes with a fork in them all around
2. Microwave them until soft. For my microwave this meant 5 minutes, then I cut them all in thirds, and microwaved again for 3 minutes. (SGT VEGAN NOTE: The pieces should cut easily with a knife. If you are wondering if they are done or not, try a piece. They should not be crunchy!!!)
3. Place all of the potatoes in the Cuisinart when ready. Add a small amount of Veganaise, with the seasoning and Earth balance.
4. Using pulse mode, blend the ingredients slowly, being sure to not to over blend. Stop the process once you reach desired consistency.
5. Serve with Earth balance spread. Tastes even better if you add roasted garlic!

♥ *Vegan Potato Salad* ♥

I used to lament how much I missed potato salad. Summer picnics just weren't the same without it. Now, no one ever has to be without potato salad again!

What you will need:

- ► Large Pot
- ► 1 lb. Bag of Potatoes
- ► Vegenaise
- ► Jar of relish
- ► Salt and Pepper to taste

What you will need to do:

1. Peel and cut potatoes into medium sized chunks
2. Place potatoes into boiling water.
3. Remove from water after potatoes begin to get soft (like el dente pasta).
4. Rinse potatoes in cold tap water.
5. After potato chunks are cold from the water, add about ½ cup Vegenaise to the potato chunks. A little more or less to taste, you want to coat it but NOT make it into Vegenaise soup.
6. Add about ¼ cup of relish
7. Enjoy!!

LEVEL UP:

If you miss the potato salad with egg in it, add about 1 cup of cold tofu scramble (minus the broccoli-use the version which includes red onion).

SOUPS

♥ *Mom's Curry Carrot Soup* ♥

What you will need:

- ► 1 large soup pot
- ► 2 lbs. carrots, peeled and quartered
- ► 1 large onion, peeled and rough chopped
- ► 1-2 tablespoons of curry powder (to taste, add more if desired)
- ► 2 quarts of vegetable broth (store bought or from vegetable bouillon cubes)
- ► cooking spray or olive oil
- ► Immersion blender

What you do:

1. Spray bottom of pot with cooking spray or add 2 T olive oil
2. Put onions and carrots in the pot, cover with the curry powder, over medium heat
3. Stir often until all is heated.
4. Add veg stock
5. Once mixture boils, turn heat down to low and cover, stirring intermittently
6. Cook for about 2 hours or until carrots are soft
7. Puree vegetables in broth with immersion blender. If you don't have an immersion blender, wait until mixture cools, then blend in regular blender.
8. Serve hot with crusty bread, or chilled with a spring of parsley

♥ *Mom's Pea Soup* ♥

What you need:

- ► 1 large soup pot (6-8 quarts)
- ► pound bag of dried peas
- ► 1 medium to large onion, peeled and chopped
- ► 1 tablespoon olive oil
- ► 2 peeled and sliced carrots
- ► 6 cups of vegetable stock (if you haven't made soup before, you can make this with vegetable bouillon cubes, just find the ones that are vegan and you are good to go)
- ► Immersion blender, vita mix, or potato masher

What you do:

1. Rinse peas in a colander, let sit and drain
2. Put olive oil in soup pot, add onions, peas, carrots and sauté on medium heat until soft
3. After 5 minutes from the time you started sautéing the onion, add the vegetable stock
4. When the mixture starts to boil, turn burner down to medium low
5. Let soup cook, stirring every 20 minutes, for about 40 minutes
6. If consistency of soup is too thick, add extra veggie broth until you are happy with it.
7. Sample soup, soup is ready when peas are totally dissolved or very soft
8. Use immersion blender, or put in vita mixer or blender, or go punk rock on it and use a potato masher.
9. Serve hot with crusty bread on a cold day or stormy night.

DESSERTS

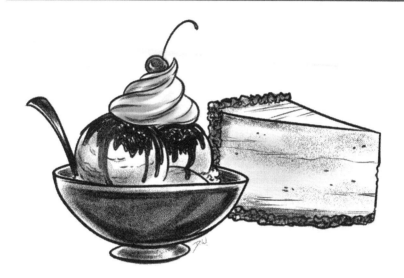

♥ *SGT Vegan's Kickass Cheesecake* ♥

Things you will need:

- ► 1 Keebler (or knock-off brand) premade graham pie crust, 6oz. Watch out for honey!!!
- ► 2 containers of Tofutti Cream Cheese 8 oz. each (other brands will work too)
- ► 1/8 cup of water
- ► 1.5 tablespoons corn starch
- ► ¾ cup of granulated sugar.

Steps:

1. Preheat oven to 350 degrees.
2. Mix sugar and cream cheese together until smooth. I like to use a Cuisinart, but a mixer will do, and if you don't have a mixer go old school with a spoon.

3. In a small bowl create a slurry by adding the cornstarch to the water.
4. Dump the slurry in with your cream cheese mixture and mix until it is even.
5. Pour the whole mixture into the pre-made pie dish.
6. Put the cheesecake in the over and bake for 1 hour, or until golden brown.
7. Take carefully out of oven. Place on counter to cool.
8. Cool completely, then put in refrigerator for several hours before serving.

LEVEL UP:
1. Chocolate Chip Cheesecake. Add a thin layer of chocolate chips (I like the Trader Joes brand ones-cheap, delicious, and accidentally vegan) on top of graham cracker crust before you put in the mixture, and then on top after the pie cools. Don't put in too many; you'll make a mess.
2. Fruit. Instead of chocolate chips, use either strawberries or blueberries on top. I feel they get messy if you add them before the cheesecake bakes.

♥ *Peanut Butter Cups* ♥

Are you angry that Reese's Peanut Butter Cups aren't vegan? Make your own, DIY!!

What you will need:
▶ 1 bag of vegan chocolate chips
▶ 1 jar of peanut butter
▶ 1 package of cupcake or candy foils
▶ cooking or baking spray (without flavor is better)

Steps:
1. Lay out foils, and spray them with baking or cooking spray.
2. Melt chocolate in a microwave safe bowl (it's easier than on the stovetop)
3. Add a layer of chocolate to the foils.

4. Add a layer of peanut butter
5. Top with a layer of chocolate
6. Chill in the refrigerator and serve. Makes a bunch!

♥ *Vegan Cinnamon Raisin Scone Recipe* ♥

My mother was a baker at a tea shop. Here is the veganized version of the scone recipe she created for me and my brother, so we could get sconed along with everyone else. Also, my mom pointed out you are going to need a kitchen scale to weigh out the ingredients to get things exact. Good Luck NOT saying "Dude, let's get sconed," when you make this.

What you need:

► parchment paper
► rolling pin
► dough cutter 2-2.25 "
► mixer with paddle attachment
► kitchen scale
► 1.5 lbs. all purpose flour
► ½ c sugar
► 2 T baking powder
► ½ tsp salt
► 1 T ENER-G egg replacer
► 6 oz. soft vegan margarine
► 6 oz. of raisins
► 2 T ground cinnamon
► 1/3 cup plus 1 T of vegan milk – coconut, soy, or almond. Your choice.

What you need to do:

1. Put mixer on stir setting and mix all dry ingredients (except raisins) for 3 minutes.
2. Add margarine, mix well.
3. Add vanilla slowly, mix well.

4. Add vegan milk slowly until mix is all moist, but not wet. This is important. The dough should feel elastic but not wet, and not lumpy. If dough still feels dry add vegan milk in 1 tsp. increments.
5. Add Raisins.
6. Knead dough, roll out on lightly floured surface. Cut with dough cutter, making a hockey puck like piece of dough. Line them up on a tray lined with parchment paper, with some space in between each scone.
7. Sprinkle unbaked scones lightly with sugar.
8. Brush tops of scones lightly with vegan milk.
9. Place tray in pre-heated center of oven.
10. Bake at 325 degrees for 25-30 minutes. Check after about 23 minutes; scones should be firm (neither hard-baked nor soft), and golden brown
11. Allow scones to cool before storing. Reheat briefly when serving.

♥ *Vegan Banana Loaf* ♥

This has become a Muir family staple. My mom's banana loaf is front and center at every family holiday brunch from Christmas to Easter and everything in between. Easy to make and freezes well.

What you will need:
▶ loaf pan or spring form pan
▶ mixer
▶ 0.5 c vegan margarine
▶ 1 c sugar
▶ 1 c mashed ripe bananas (about 1.5 medium bananas)
▶ 4 T of water
▶ 2 c all purpose flour
▶ 1 tsp baking soda
▶ 1 tsp cinnamon
▶ 0.5 tsp salt

What you do:

1. Grease baking pan with Crisco all vegetable shortening, or use cooking spray
2. Fill pans about halfway with mixture.
3. Bake at 350 for 45-60 minutes. Toothpick test for doneness- toothpick should come out clean. Baking time varies on type of pan you use. If you use spring form pan or wide pan it will be done sooner, and if you use narrow loaf pan it will take a little longer.

LEVEL UP:

Add chopped walnuts and raisins, and/or 1 tsp. of orange peel zest.

♥ *Coconut Ice Cream* ♥

When I was in vegan culinary school I made ice cream often, as store bought vegan ice cream was in scarce supply back then. Luckily, this ice cream recipe is made with items you can easily purchase at any grocery store chain in America, and the ice cream maker can be bought at almost any department store. While there are many delicious store bought vegan brands of ice cream available at time of writing, making your own ice cream is fun and vegan delicious!

Please make sure you get the canned coconut milk with a high fat content, not the Coconut Milk you put on your cereal. What makes ice cream recipe work is a high fat and sugar content, and you don't want to cheat yourself of that. Please also recognize the more expensive ice cream makers are going to work a lot better than the cheap ones, but the end result tastes about the same. Just don't gobble the whole thing down in one sitting and you'll be all right. This recipe makes about two pints of ice cream.

What you will need:

- ► electric ice cream maker
- ► 1 cup of vegan granulated sugar
- ► 0.5 cup of water, or coffee if you are making coffee flavor
- ► 3.5 cups of coconut milk. The canned stuff, with lots of fat, not the stuff you put on your cereal

What you do:

In a pot, heat the sugar and water and make a thick syrup, stirring to make sure it doesn't burn. When the syrup is thick enough to coat a spoon, remove from heat and cool. Cool the mixture down, and throw in the coconut milk and the other parts of the recipe into the container part of the ice cream maker. From there follow whatever the ice cream maker instructions say to do, which should be about an hour of churning. Then put the mixer into the freezer to get really cold.

LEVEL UP:

Add a small handful of chocolate chips for chocolate chip ice cream. For more coconut taste, add sweetened shredded coconut. If you want to do coffee ice cream, add the cold brewed coffee as mentioned above, and then mix in ½ tsp of coffee grounds into the mixture for real coffee flavor.

♥ *Banana Ice Cream* ♥

I'm not sure how this is scientifically possible, but blended frozen bananas create a perfect dessert treat similar to soft serve. It is quicker to make than coconut ice cream, with a lot less fat. Enjoy!!

What you will need:

- ► Cuisinart food processor
- ► 4-6 frozen bananas (let thaw 15 minutes)
- ► 1 T vegan cocoa powder

What you do:

Simply put the bananas in the food processor, add cocoa powder, and mix until blended. Serve any way you want, but not with bananas on top. That would be bananas!!

Alternate Idea:

Instead of coca powder, add a handful of strawberries for strawberry ice cream.

Chapter 19

7 Days of Vegan Food

ONE OF THE BIGGEST BARRIERS people have in becoming vegan is the fear of just not knowing what to eat. I hope this chapter will give you some ideas on what to make for yourself, and show you just how easy being vegan is in the 21ˢᵗ century. Besides these menu ideas, I suggest always having Cliff Bars or other vegan snacks on hand, thus making life easy and taking the pressure off of you to find food. Please adjust this menu according to your own caloric needs. These food suggestions are for the average-sized person with an active lifestyle, NOT for someone trying to lose weight.

Please note the importance of having vegetables as the main attraction of every meal. Yes, it is awesome that we now have vegan cheese, and I'm very happy protein substitutes are available at practically every regular supermarket in America. However, vegetables should always be the most important part of every healthy meal, so make sure you don't forget to give them a big spot on your plate. Just because you can now find vegan junk food everywhere doesn't mean you should eat it.

In addition to this, other than a small, 6 oz. glass of juice with breakfast, I suggest making water your beverage of choice with every meal. I also drink black coffee, both because I work nights and because I am a Veteran. (SGT VEGAN NOTE: Drinking your coffee black also means it is a zero calorie beverage). If you follow this pattern, make sure you don't over do. Excess caffeine intake can cause insomnia and GI issues.

I also highly recommend healthy snacking between meals. Carrots, fruit, protein bars. Eat as much fruit or vegetables as you want (unless you are on a restrictive diet), but take it easy on the protein bars.

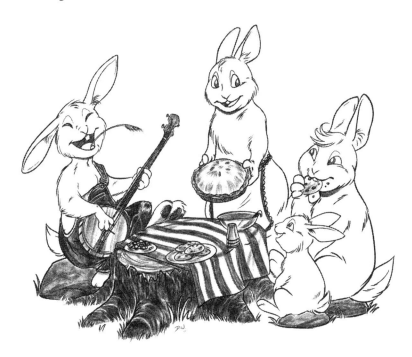

Day1: Monday

Breakfast: Tofu Scramble, English Muffin (Trader Joes has a vegan one), orange juice, coffee or tea

Lunch: Tofurkey Wrap (4 Tofurkey slices on your favorite burrito wrap with fresh spinach, tomato, Vegenaise, Sriracha, and avocado) carrots and hummus, and an apple

Snack: Vegan yogurt, mix in a package of raisins and nuts

Dinner: Spaghetti and Tofurkey Italian Sausage, small piece of garlic bread, cup of steamed broccoli, side salad

Day 2: Tuesday

Breakfast: Bowl of steel cut oats with almond or soy milk and fruit, cup of juice, coffee or tea

Lunch: 2 Veggie Hotdogs Litelife or other brand), apple slices, cold beverage

Snack: Granola Bar and piece of fruit

Dinner: Seitan steak cutlets, grilled asparagus spears, mashed potatoes, gravy, side salad.

Day 3: Wednesday

Breakfast: Bagel, Tofutti cream cheese, jelly, coffee, juice, fruit cup

Lunch: Dr. Preggers Ramen soup, carrot sticks and hummus

Snack: Dried Fruit Mix, piece of fruit

Dinner: Bowel of Chili, corn bread, cup of rice, side salad

Day 4: Thursday

Breakfast: Soyrizo with tofu scramble and an English Muffin

Lunch: Veggie Burger, single serving of vegan mac n cheese, vegetable, salad, beverage

Snack: Bananas and peanut butter sandwich, fruit salad

Dinner: Vegan Sir Fry with Gardein Orange Chicken, broccoli, rice, side salad

Day 5: Friday

Breakfast: Waffles, Gardein chicken, coffee
Lunch: Vegan Sushi Rolls, cold green tea
Snack: protein shake or fruit smoothie
Dinner: Vegan Pizza! Beverage, salad, cooked veggie of your
  choice

Day 6: Saturday

Breakfast: Tofu Mc Muffin, orange juice
Lunch: BBQ tempeh sandwich, couscous, vegetable
Snack: peanut butter pretzels, piece of fruit
Dinner: Stuffed Shells, garlic bread, cooked broccoli

Day 7: Sunday

Brunch: Pancakes, tofu scramble, soy sausage patty, maple
  syrup
Lunch: Vegan Fajitas, Mexican Rice, avocado, beverage
Snack: smoothie with banana, fruit, vegan milk of choice
Dinner: Good Shepard's Pie, salad, cooked veggie of your
  choice

Chapter 20

Eating Vegan on the Cheap

ONE COMMON MISCONCEPTION about being vegan is that it is more expensive than being a meat eater. Like every myth, this one is also false, and I am here to set the record straight.

First let's consider the source of the myth. Because Animal Agriculture is heavily subsidized by the government, hamburgers are usually going to be cheaper than veggie burgers (SGT VEGAN NOTE: Except for McDonald's in India, where they cost less than one dollar each). Additionally, buying fancy, "organic", vegan products in high-end super markets like Whole Foods (often dubbed "Whole Paycheck") can be more expensive than a similar animal-sourced version at a regular supermarket chain.

While this may be the case, it doesn't mean being vegan is inherently more expensive than being a meat eater. Comparing vegans who shop at Whole Foods to meat eaters who shop at regular supermarkets is like comparing apples to Oreos. Instead, how about comparing people who shop at the same supermarket? Many meat eaters also shop at Whole Foods, and they aren't exactly saving money by buying their meat there. If we compare vegans who shop at Whole Foods with meat eating yuppies who also shop there, you will find that both groups spend a lot of money on groceries.

When it comes to comparing vegans to meat eaters who shop at "regular" supermarket chains, you will again find they also spend about the same. The only difference might be some "regular" supermarket chains charge more for processed vegan foods (like meat and milk substitutes), so if you buy them there, you might end up going over budget. Solution: only buy those products when they are on sale, or at Trader Joes, where they are usually a little cheaper, or make your own (see the cooking section of this book for details on making a meat substitute called "seitan").

If you take the sometimes pricey processed vegan treats out of the equation, being vegan can actually be quite cheaper than eating the Standard American Diet. Vegetables and other produce are usually inexpensive, as are old school vegan protein staples like tofu, peanut butter, and beans. A lot of healthy, delicious, vegan dishes can be made for next to nothing, and rice or other grains can be bought in bulk. No one ever went broke eating rice and beans, pasta, or tofu stir-fry. Being vegan does not have to be expensive. Hopefully this chapter can give you some ideas to help you get the most bang for your vegan bucks.

Tips for being vegan on the cheap:

1. Save going out to eat for special occasions. For the budget-minded individual this is a no-brainer, but we aren't all like that. Restaurants are almost always going to be more expensive than cooking for yourself. If you do go to a restaurant, avoid buying things like drinks (just empty calories and a waste of money anyway), and unless it is something awesome you can't make for yourself at home, avoid dessert.

2. Learn to cook. Consider this your invitation to learn. Not only is cooking your own meals cheaper, it has been shown to be healthier as well.

3. Limit your shopping in Whole Foods, and other specialty markets. Notice I didn't say not to go there at all. I think Whole Foods has a lot of great products, and some of

them are actually reasonably priced. Occasionally their meat- alternative products will actually be cheaper than if you bought them at "regular" supermarkets. So limit your shopping there to specialty items, and only get the ones there that are reasonably priced.

4. Don't look down on Dollar Store food. There are some great deals to be had, and the produce can be very affordable. Sometimes you can even buy soy milk there.

5. Farmer's Markets are great, just not the ones in yuppie areas. I live in Culver City CA, so for me, "Farmer's Markets" are usually super expensive. Where I grew up in PA, though, they had a place called "Produce Junction," which was a farmer's market for normal people, and those prices were great. See what is available in your area and shop accordingly.

6. Eat lots of vegetables! I get some people have a need to eat only organic produce, but let's face it, since "organic" is now a buzz word, it is often more expensive to buy organic vegetables, and sometimes not even worth it. If two vegetables are equally priced, go for the organic one. If you find organic to be too expensive, then don't buy organic. In the long run you are still better off with eating non- organic vegetables than not eating vegetables at all. If you are wondering which fruits and vegetables are most important to buy organic certified, do a GOOGLE search for "Dirty Dozen organic list."

7. While fresh vegetables are awesome, I am never afraid to buy frozen or canned vegetables. Sometimes the convenience of cooking with them makes up for them not being fresh, and of course they are usually cheaper, too.

How I shop:

I buy a lot of my staples at Trader Joe's, as they are reasonably priced. I get the rest of my food at either the "regular" supermarket when they have sales, or at a store called Sprout's, which also has a lot of sales. I only buy ice cream and other "luxury" items when there is a sale, and I try to avoid junk food, vegan or otherwise.

Vegetables should always be the main part of every healthy vegan diet, and they themselves are usually not expensive unless you are buying exotic, rare vegetables. I was vegan for many years before it "got cool" and had to get by without fancy vegan substitute meats, ice cream, or junk food. Whole Foods Market wasn't around back then either. You can easily be vegan without spending a lot of money.

Remember, there are many dishes that can be made cheaply. Pasta is always a delicious vegan staple. Tacos and burritos are cheap and easy to make vegan, and rice and beans should be a healthy staple of anyone's daily intake. Beans themselves, whether canned or rehydrated, are a cheap and delicious source of protein and fiber. You are only limited by your creativity in the kitchen.

Chapter 21

So You Want to Open a Vegan Restaurant?

A LOT OF PEOPLE CONSIDER completely changing the direction of their lives after they open their eyes to the suffering of animals. One of the most tangible forms of "economic direct action" you can take to save animals is opening a vegan restaurant. The following is an interview with the owner and operator of Philadelphia's Blackbird Pizzeria, Mark Mebus.

Mark, how long have you been vegan, and what inspired that change?

I have been vegan since 1998. I went vegan because I was unhappy with how animals are exploited in industrialized society, whether in eating meat and animal products such as dairy or eggs, or wearing their skins such as leather and fur. Once my eyes were opened to that reality I decided that I wanted to be as far from supporting that exploitation as possible. It was a rather quick transition for me, about 4-5 months from meat-eater to vegetarian to vegan.

Has being vegan influenced the direction that your life has gone in?

Entirely. It's been the basis of my culinary career and opening a business. Being vegan has probably influenced my life more than any other decision I have ever made.

How long have you been in business?

I opened Blackbird Pizzeria on September 30, 2010.

How did you come up with the name and concept?

Blackbird Pizzeria gets its name from a Beatles song that I used to sing to my daughter when she was a baby. The concept of opening a vegan pizzeria came from pizza being the most important food on the planet. (SGT VEGAN NOTE: Goddamn Right!) I talked to a lot of people before I opened Blackbird. In these conversations it came out time and time again that the main thing that kept people from being vegan was lack of access to vegan pizza. I wanted to create a space that would be causal and enjoyable and get more people to eat healthy and save animals. Since "lack of pizza" was what was keeping a lot of people from going vegan, I decided to tackle that pizza problem head on with Blackbird Pizzeria.

What kind of experience is necessary in order to start a restaurant?

I think it is good to work for at least 2 years at a restaurant to see how it operates before opening your own. If you were opening a quick service vegan burger joint, maybe only 2 years' experience would be necessary, but for a higher end restaurant it could possibly take up to 10 years to get the experience that you need to be successful.

Do you need to go to culinary school to open a restaurant?

I have mixed feelings about that. If you want a cooking career, a culinary degree will help you to get your foot in the door, but I wouldn't call it necessary. As far as owning a restaurant goes, it all depends on what you will be serving in your restaurant. For me, I already had a culinary background, so I knew what I was doing. You don't have to be a culinary mastermind to open a restaurant; you just need to work with someone who is. If you don't know how to cook, you can always hire a consultant. I knew how to cook, so I didn't have to.

Is it more important to get cooking or managerial experience for opening a restaurant?

Knowing how to run a restaurant can be more important than knowing how to cook. Again, you can always hire someone to cook. The biggest factor in running a successful restaurant is knowing how to manage costs, specifically balancing labor and food costs. I've known excellent chefs who have opened their own restaurants and had to close them as well. Being able to manage those costs is the key to success.

What are the steps to opening a restaurant?

The first step is to write a business plan. Once you have a solid concept of what you want to do and how you want to do it, look for funding to make it all happen. It can cost anywhere from 70-350 thousand dollars to open a restaurant. That money can either come from investors, or loans. The amount of money you will need depends on what your concept is, what you will be cooking, and where you want to open a restaurant. The same restaurant will cost differently depending on where you are opening it. Once you have secured finances and find your location, you can get started on your build-out. Of course, using the existing apparatus of a place that is already built like a restaurant will save you a lot of start-up money. It can all be a lengthy process, taking anywhere from 3-6 months to get your space ready for you to start cooking and accepting customers. In Blackbird's case, we were lucky in opening the restaurant because we found an establishment that was already a pizza place, so we didn't have to spend the extra money creating one. We got the money from friends and family and were able to fully fund it without taking out bank loans.

Any advice for vegans starting their own restaurant?

There is a lot to deal with when you first open a restaurant. The most important thing that you can do to set yourself up for success is to know the ins and outs of the industry by having adequate hands-on experience. The restaurant industry is a difficult and rewarding business to be in, but too many people rush in without having the proper knowledge and experience. You wear too many hats as a restaurant owner to just "wing it." The more experience that you have, the higher your chances are for success. Also, when opening a new business, you will want to have a decent financial buffer to weather the highs and lows. You should aim to keep 3-6 months' worth of operating costs in reserve for the first year or so if you can.

Mark, what are your favorite Philadelphia area restaurants?

In my opinion, the TOP 3 vegan places in the Philly area are: V Street (a street food restaurant from the creators of Vedge), Sprig and Vine (My friend Ross' place in the Philly burbs) and Vedge. The owner of Vedge, Rich Landau, had a lot to do with bringing mainstream attention to vegan food just by having restaurants that were so damn good. When Rich moved Horizons from the Philly suburbs to the city, it caused veganism to explode. (SGT VEGAN NOTE: Horizons is still one of my favorite vegan restaurants ever.) Nowadays Philly is out of control, and there are new vegan spots opening up all the time! More and more people are going vegan, as the importance of being vegan becomes mainstream and is backed by science. We need to eat healthier AND protect the environment at the same time. Even among people who won't completely embrace a vegan lifestyle, there is interest in eating vegan food these days. When people see that vegan restaurants can be financially successful, they make other restaurants want to serve vegan food in order to cash in on the niche market that already exists. Right now so many people -— not even just vegans, but vegetarians and omnivores as well --will check out your restaurant when they hear it is vegan, and there will be interest EVEN BEFORE YOU OPEN! Vegan is not a turn off anymore. It is the future.

You can find out more about the best Pizza Place in America at www.blackbirdpizzeria.com. **Congratulations Blackbird Pizzeria for being voted the Best Philly Vegan Cheesesteak twice in a row!**

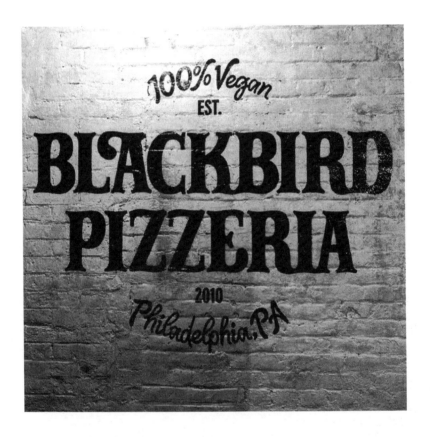

Part 4

VEGAN PEOPLE

THE FOLLOWING IS A COLLECTION of interviews. Some of the interviews were done over the phone, some via email, and some in person. My criteria for choosing who to interview was the following:

1. Must have been vegan for at least 2 YEARS
2. Must be doing something interesting with their lives

I chose to interview people from all walks of life: health care, law enforcement, chefs, lawyers, athletes, students, and musicians. These are people living active, healthy lives, fueled only by plants and a love of animals. The stereotype of vegans being lazy hippies ended a long time ago. Welcome to the Next Generation of Veganism!

Questions:

1. Name, occupation?
2. How long have you been vegan?
3. How did you become vegan and why are you still vegan?
4. How has being vegan changed your life?
5. Tell me about something cool that you've done.
6. Advice for new vegans?
7. Favorite recipe/ restaurant?

LAURIE WISOTSKY

Surgery PA and competitive short distance runner

How long have you been vegan?

I slowly entertained the idea of becoming vegan in early 2013. By summer of that year I was making small changes to become vegan. And by the end of the year I was totally vegan.

Why did you become vegan?

I became vegan because I did not like how I was feeling. I always felt bloated; I was moody and just felt worn down. I used to excuse how I was feeling by contributing it to hard training and just life with two busy kids. I was tired of feeling that way and finally decided to make a change. I did lots of research and talked extensively to healthcare professionals about the vegan lifestyle and healthier living in general. Initially I was totally opposed to going vegan. I told my nutritionist, "I don't want to be that girl who goes to a party and there isn't anything I can eat, or my friends don't know what to do with me." So I became "veganish" as I called it and just eliminated dairy and red meat. I also went totally organic. I liked the results I was seeing just on those small changes so I decided to go "full-on" vegan. I'm still vegan because I am feeling the best I have ever felt! Also, as a competitive athlete, I am performing stronger than I ever have.

How has being vegan changed your life?

I'm a happier person in general which has spilled over into all aspects of my life. As a result, I have had many exciting opportunities and experiences.

Tell us about something cool that you've done?

I did medical missions for a bit in Guatemala. It was the most rewarding experience of my life. I would travel to Guatemala with a team of healthcare professionals for a week. We would perform surgeries on the people from the rural villages in Guatemala. They were so kind and grateful for all of our help.

Advice for new vegans?

My advice to new vegans is to be patient with the process of transitioning. Our palates in general are used to all the sugar, fat, and grease that's in the usual American diet, so initially vegan dishes may not taste as flavorful or satisfying. But they are! I found it took time to get my palate used to eating a plant-based diet. The other piece of advice I would give is to transition slowly. Being vegan is on the extreme spectrum of eating so eliminating everything at once will feel overwhelming. Also, take the time to read the labels on food packages and don't be afraid to ask servers at a restaurant what's in your food, dressing, or sauces. Many times restaurants can accommodate you and make a vegan dish.

Favorite recipes?

I have a lot favorite recipes. I get many from the *Oh She Glows* cookbook. They are very easy and don't take a lot of time to prepare. I also love the recipes from *One Green Planet*.

DARREN YOUNG

Executive Director of Sammy's Hope
President of 'For This One'
Partner/Owner Tekpro Systems LLC

How long have you been vegan?

I went vegetarian in 1989, vegan in 1991.

How/why did you go vegan and why are you still vegan?

I started the vegetarian thing my senior year in high school, December 1989. I was in the skate and hardcore scene, so I was aware of the vegetarian straight edge thing, but didn't know anyone vegetarian personally.

One night lying in bed, I had a very simple and obvious thought. "Those are fucking animals, man; I'm not doing that anymore." That was pretty much it for meat, other than some fish my mother insisted on in order for me not to die, which I phased out within the first six months or so.

I had never really considered the vegan thing until I met a couple of people who were vegan my first year away at college as a photography major in the Fall of 1991. It made me consider the cruelty of subjecting an animal to a life of suffering. I didn't eat animals, because I didn't want animals killed on my behalf, but it was almost worse to realize that other animals were still being forced to endure a lifetime of suffering on my behalf.

The environmental and health benefits that go along with being vegan are also important to me, but the main reason for my being vegan will always be about not being a part of the cruelty and suffering associated with non-vegan diets.

How has being vegan changed your life?

Well, the most obvious thing is that I have become very involved in animal welfare as an adult, but I think there is something less obvious worth looking at too.

Coming up in the skate and hardcore/punk scene at the time I did, I guess I made some choices that other teenagers didn't. Instead of going to the mall with a bunch of friends, I was going to hardcore shows getting kicked in the head. These are certainly very different ways to spend one's time, but both are mostly choices of personal preference. I think the difference with the choice to go veg and eventually vegan was that these were truly moral choices that went against normal conventions, not just personal preferences that were generally discouraged.

I think this tendency to consider things outside of normal conventions led to my wife and I leaving well-paying jobs to start our own computer consulting business. Where it gets interesting is when we used our experience running our business to co-found two non-profit organizations. 'For This One' was started in 2009 to do aid work in Haiti and 'Sammy's Hope' (sammyshope.org) was started in 2010 to do animal welfare work in our community. In January 2015, Sammy's Hope opened its own animal shelter, the Sammy's Hope Animal Welfare and Adoption Center. Currently both me and my wife are working full-time for a national animal welfare organization doing behavior work with dogs from cruelty cases.

So, the whole hardcore music thing led to the vegan thing both directly and indirectly in much the same way quitting the corporate world led to starting non-profit organizations. In both cases, doing generally unconventional things I wanted to do personally and the experiences that came along with that led to doing things I felt compelled to do morally that I may not have had the courage to do otherwise.

Tell me about something cool that you've done.

When volunteering in Haiti, I find the grumpiest, most jaded kids wherever we happen to be for the week and make them smile before we leave. Sometimes it takes just about the whole week, but I have pulled it off every time so far and they are my favorite kids there. That is something cool that I have done, and if you ever get the chance, I highly recommend it!

Advice for new vegans?

You will need to cook for yourself a lot. I think it is important to learn easy and quick ways to cook fresh vegetables. Learning how to steam or fry vegetables like carrots, cauliflower, and broccoli, and how to sauté leafy greens with garlic or onions is a great start. Also learn some very simple recipes with foods like tofu, beans (canned beans are fine), and quinoa. It's probably good to start out by limiting yourself to 4 ingredients per recipe plus some spices. Don't make eating healthy too complicated. Unless you have plenty of free time and really enjoy cooking, save the big fancy recipes for special occasions.

Favorite recipe?

A current favorite is Afghan Pumpkin. Sautéed pumpkin simmered in a sweet tomato, garlic, ginger, and cilantro sauce.

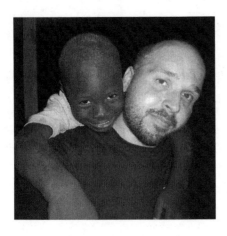

Darren Young on Haiti Mission Trip, 2010. Photo courtesy of Darren Young

CARRIE

Attorney

How long have you been vegan?

I have been vegan since 2012.

How/why did you go vegan and why are you still vegan?

I went vegetarian in 1997 after watching a documentary on PBS about how marine parks got their orcas. In 2009, I received a flyer regarding "free range" eggs and milk. It planted a seed for sure. After my boyfriend and I broke up in 2012, I started going to Vegan Meetup events. One gal I randomly met grew up on a small dairy farm. She told me about how the cows were impregnated continuously to keep the milk flowing and how the male calves were killed, or sold for veal and then killed. She discussed some of the husbandry practices and/or abuse she witnessed. I never ate dairy again. I stopped eating eggs too, although I didn't find out about the horrid life of hens until I visited a farm sanctuary called "Animal Place." I have never since seen the gal who told me her dairy farm experiences. I'm not sure if she knows how influential she was in my decision to transition to a vegan lifestyle. I stay vegan mostly out of a spiritual commitment.

How has being vegan changed your life?

Probably the biggest change has been my persistent advocacy of the moral, environmental, and nutritional benefits of a vegan lifestyle. I can discuss and cite studies or references regarding any of these topics off the top of my head. To support this effort, I took the Cornell plant-based nutrition course a few years back. I still stay up to date on nutritional studies. I have a strong spiritual commitment to nonviolence toward animals in addition to a moral, and intellectual commitment. I have never understood what a spiritual commitment was prior to being vegan despite growing up Catholic. I've never been a religious person, and I don't feel comfortable assuming there is a God. But even if I did, finding a spiritual home would be tough, and it saddens me that even most "do no harm" Buddhists are not vegan. So to compensate for this void, almost all of my friends are vegan. When I first was vegan, I found another vegan interested in building community. We would go to events, actively collect names of people we met and friend them on Facebook, and then invite them to various events. The result of these efforts has provided a strong inner circle of local vegan friends.

Tell me about something cool that you've done.

Personally, I think the coolest thing I've done is put myself through school (with a huge assist from the State of California) then studying for and passing the bar. Now I work quite productively at the State Department of Public Health and I love that I repaid that debt and then some. But most people think what's coolest are my vacations. In my undergrad at UCLA, I worked at National Parks during the summer (Grand Tetons, Glacier, Sequoia, Lake Powell), a few ski resorts in the winter (Breckenridge, Diamond Peak.) I more recently have taken my vacations at surf camps (Bali, Costa Rica, Mexico, Nicaragua, Australia.) I am planning my next one in Barbados at a raw food surf camp.

Advice for new vegans?

Take vegan cooking courses, meet other vegans, and stay tuned into the animal suffering you are preventing. Even if you can't be an "activist," just modeling a fun vegan lifestyle is very persuasive to others.

MILO IMRIE

Veterinary Assistant, former Marine

How long have you been vegan?

I have been vegan since mid-February of 2014

How/why did you go vegan and why are you still vegan?

I was being held in administrative segregation in the San Mateo County Jail in Redwood City, California. The menu was not very varied, and the lack of other stimulation made me focus on food for my sense of well-being. There was a decent variety of breakfast and dinners, but lunch everyday was a baloney sandwich, and I hated baloney. One day I noticed that the guy in the cell next to me was getting hummus, GRAPES and cheese with regularity. I said "Hey man, how do you get hummus all the damn time?" He said "I'm Jewish, and this is the kosher diet." I requested a vegetarian diet immediately.

I noticed that my bouts of diarrhea and vomiting seemed to lessen. I also noticed that I didn't miss the shitty meat at all; I was fine with beans and the like. So, the door to questioning what I had been fed my whole life had less monsters on the other side of it. I made the observation that we prisoners were living much like the animals that were farmed for the products I had now forsaken. I knew I had reason to be there in a cage, and couldn't come up with any better way for society to deal with me in my current state, so I was ok with it. The pigs and cows though... they did nothing wrong. They were born into suffering and slavery. Indeed, even the phrase that first comes to mind to describe inhumane treatment throughout the ages --

"they treated us like animals!" -- became a little curious. Why are we treating the animals so poorly?

So I was bailed out as a vegetarian. I stuck with it. Why not, after all, as I had gotten fat from inactivity and it seemed a helpful habit in order to trim down again.

The coup-de-grace was a woman whom I liked. She gave me a book called *Farm Sanctuary*, about an organization built largely on the initiative of a man named Gene Bauer. Mr. Bauer had brass balls and was vegan before it was cool. He put a lot of life into fighting for animal rights laws and ironically making great strides for the safety of commercial meat products in America. Farm Sanctuary now has several locations across the country where they tend to the livelihoods of rescued farm animals. It's the most noble, good thing that I can imagine. One of the most important realizations he triggered was that pigs are emotionally and intellectually on the same level as dogs, possibly even higher, and yet we treat dogs like princes, and we condemn pigs to death. I was vegan before I finished the introduction to the book and haven't looked back since. I am not paying for the way they treat animals and what ranching does to the planet. Not my dollars, not my votes.

How has being vegan changed your life?

Honestly, not as much as I would have expected. It does become something you have to be socially prepared for. People who have not been exposed to our kind will immediately re-frame their perception of you. You will encounter a barrage of stereotypes and myths from everyone you meet, and foolish "advice" from the well-intentioned. You'll get cookbooks for Christmas and birthdays forever unless you put the kibosh on it amongst your family. "How vegan" you are and why you are vegan will also influence your interactions with other vegans as well.

Tell me about something cool that you've done.

I helped convince one of the Veterinarians whom I work with to go vegan for a couple months and have influenced my family to eat cruelty-free meals around holidays. Even those small things have a calculable impact on water consumption and ending cruelty. I recently made a commitment to give 10% of my net income to charitable causes. One of my favorites is Apropos, which is a project that trains African Pouched Rats to detect landmines. That may not seem vegan on the surface, but I honestly see it as species uplift, practically Promethean, the way they do it. The rats are too small to set off landmines and have some of the most sensitive noses in the mammalian kingdom. They are also highly trainable, and are much cheaper to feed and easier to handle than dogs. They are raised or bred and selected and trained and eventually have an excellent success ratio for picking even extremely old explosives out of long taboo landscapes. I am assured they have a comfortable retirement when they can no longer serve. To me, that is essentially citizenship, doing the best we can possibly do for the animals among us. They may be humble rats, but they have a noble place in the Federation of Earth! Seriously they have cleared huge areas that used to take the limbs off of little kids. If I was a rat, I can't imagine a higher aspiration; I would want to be a bomb-sniffing rat. Golden Rule test passed.

Advice for new vegans?

It's not a diet; it's a philosophy. If you're doing it to be skinny or healthy or hip you are a fake and a flake and you'll fail. Do it because you don't want to be responsible for evil. Don't start unless you intend to finish. Ignore the magical meat substitutes and weird fancy fake cheeses. They are delicious, and I do miss quesadillas. You can eat those things when you go out to a restaurant. For yourself, learn to eat healthy and vegan and cheap from your local supermarket. Let the people see your cart overflowing with kale, potatoes, and beans, for verily I say unto you such simple things and some rosemary are all you need. Don't wear leather, not even fake leather. Same with fake fur. It looks like real leather to anyone who isn't obsessed with such things and it continues to normalize the wearing of the flesh of other creatures. Isn't that kind of weird? Don't be too friendly to "well, I'm vegetarians." They're frauds and they know it, unless they are trying to be vegan and in a tough spot with their family. The hunger lasts a year. Sorry, no bones about it (pun not intended but I like it). You might crave things you can't put a name to, for reasons you don't really understand. It can be rough, no lie, and a lot of us end up as "carbaholics" for a time to compensate. You might get skinny and then a little fat for a time. You won't have any negative health effects as long as you get adequate iron and adequate vitamin C to process it. You will probably need a b12 supplement as well, and it is cheaper than your bad habits I promise. I donate platelets every other week and don't do any weird dietary supplements and my hemoglobin levels are fine. True, I am a robust white caveman, but I believe this is possible for all. You're on the right path. Don't quit. Think about what a difference you are now making just by living what you believe in. When it gets hard or you get lonely, then is the time to watch some good vegan propaganda and get the good numbers back in your head. With that in mind...there are some nuts among us. Don't let them give us a bad name by being overly aggressive, obnoxious, or the WORST thing, dishonest. No lies about superhuman disease curing miracles of the vegan diet, that's bullshit. Yeah it is often healthier, but only if done properly, just like "regular" eating. It did do wonders for my cardio though, no lie. I think I now have lower cholesterol but I don't know for sure. It will come up in conversation almost immediately and people will act like you bring it up all the time. Really, you are just saying no to the ice cream. Try to just say no without saying your vegan unless you're pressed on it. And don't bring it up unless asked. But when they ask, PREACH!

Favorite restaurants?

Oh man, the fact that this is hard to answer is a big part of why I love Los Angeles! I think I have to go with Araya's Place, which happens to be one of the top-rated Thai places in LA on its own merits. They have a pumpkin curry that is divine. However, if a non-vegan is visiting, I take them to Vegan Glory. It's right down the street but a much more casual atmosphere. The name is so in-your-face it sets them up to be uncomfortable, but the restaurant itself is casual, full of natural light, recently and tastefully remodeled, and doesn't spit vegan at you at all! They are put at ease. The menu unapologetically says "Beef Jerky" and "Chicken Satay" and the like, and those two things are what I always get newcomers because they are the most intoxicating not-meat dishes I have ever had. Vegan Glory has gotten great reviews, people love it, and every bite is vegan!

WHITNEY LAURITSEN

Vegan content creator and entrepreneur

How long have you been vegan?

I've been vegan since fall 2003.

How/why did you go vegan and why are you still vegan?

I went vegetarian in 2003 because I was inspired by a friend. Then six months later, after doing lots of research and experiencing all the joy of giving up meat, I went vegan. My preliminary motivation was centered around health, and over the years I fell in love with the lifestyle because of how good I felt, emotionally, physically and spiritually. It's fun discovering new ways to be eco-friendly, healthy and compassionate!

How has being vegan changed your life?

Being vegan has given me a whole new outlook on life. I feel more connected to my body and the planet. I'm so much healthier, especially since I started eating a whole- foods diet. Growing up, I always felt really out of control with food, and all I really knew was to watch out for fat and calorie content, so I couldn't understand why I didn't feel or look good. When I went vegetarian I felt an immediate difference, which has continued to blossom as I've modified my diet to be healthier over the years. I lost weight, my skin looks great, I have tons of energy, my digestion has improved, and I rarely get sick. I feel in control now because I understand what foods are good for my body and why.

My career has also been shaped by my vegan lifestyle. I started my website because of my passion for the lifestyle and it turned into my full-time focus.

Tell me about something cool that you've done.

In 2013 I made a vegan B.L.T. while skydiving. I always wanted to incorporate skydiving into one of my YouTube videos and thought what better way than to make a recipe in the sky! I jumped out of plane with a fanny pack full of tempeh bacon, lettuce, tomato, Vegenaise and a tortilla, then put it all together once under a deployed parachute canopy in the air. Definitely one of the coolest things I've ever done!

Advice for new vegans?

You can do it! It may sound cheesy, but the most common thing I hear from people is, "I could never do that." It took me a while to get to this point, but it happened because I never told myself that I couldn't do it. It's also important to be patient and open – know that few things happen overnight and always be willing to change your mind. You will meet many people with lots of opinions on health and wellness – listen to what they have to say, then take time to research it on your own to see if you agree. All of the information will lead you to discovering what works best for you, and though the road may be bumpy at times, never give up!

Favorite recipe/ restaurant?

Millennium in the Bay Area is my favorite vegan restaurant of all time. When I found out that they had to close their original location in San Francisco, I literally got teary eyed and changed my plans so I could dine there before they closed. I was so relieved to hear that they are opening a new location in the East Bay. Their food is outstanding and I love the atmosphere too. I can't say that I have a favorite recipe because I'm not much of a chef and my food preferences change a lot. But my favorite meal to make at home is a rice bowl with vegetables. I change up the veggies and the sauces almost every time I make it, all depending on my mood.

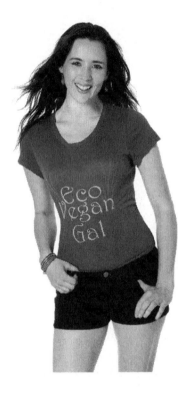

The Eco-Vegan Gal, photo courtesy of Whitney Lauritsen.

Michael Cavanaugh

Reliability engineer

How long have you been vegan?

I've been vegan since 2004.

Why did you go vegan?

Out of ethical concerns for how animals are treated at factory farms etc.

How has being vegan changed your life?

It has had a large impact on my philosophy in general. I feel that I am a better person as I think I am more considerate of others, both human and all other life forms. I also feel a greater connection to the environment and the resources that we use and often abuse.

Tell me about something cool that you've done.

I went stand up paddle boarding for the first time the other day. It was fun and it was easier than I thought it would be.

Any advice for new vegans?

Don't sweat the little things.

Favorite restaurant or recipe?

In the South Bay of Los Angeles, there is a cool place called The Green Temple that I like. Even though it is just a vegetarian restaurant, most dishes are easily veganized.

Mike's Chili Recipe

Grab a big ass cooking pot, fill it around 1/3 full with water, add 1 cup of lentils and turn on the heat. Chop up whatever vegetables you plan to use. I usually use peppers, tomatoes, onions, garlic, and cucumber. After the lentils have cooked for about 45 minutes, add a cup of rice, and a cup of quinoa. Prepare the spice mix. I never measure any of this stuff. I do it by feel so it's a bit different every time. I use masala mixes that can be obtained at any grocery store along with whatever else I feel like throwing into the mix. Usually it's a combination of: ground pepper, cumin seeds, curry powder, garam masala, maybe chana masala, maybe coriander, maybe turmeric, maybe some biryani spice mix. It depends how I feel. By the way, I never use any salt or sugar in anything I make and you shouldn't either if you know what's good for you. After the rice and quinoa have cooked for ~15 minutes add the vegetables and spice mix. You can add more water depending on what consistency you want. I prefer a thick consistency. Stir it up well and check the spiciness, add more spices if you feel the need. If it's too spicy then "man up" and eat it anyway. Let the pot simmer for another 5 minutes or so then turn off fire and let it cool and you're ready to rock and roll!

HEATHER SHENKMAN

Interventional Cardiologist

How long have you been vegan?

I have been vegan since 2005.

How/why did you go vegan and why are you still vegan?

I went vegan for the animals and because plant-based diets reverse the diseases that I treat as a cardiologist.

How has being vegan changed your life?

Being vegan has helped me to be more holistic in my approach to patient care. While medicines are an important part of cardiac care, I focus on lifestyle-- diet, exercise, maintaining a healthy weight, and managing stress.

Tell me about something cool that you've done.

I am a competitive triathlete. In 2013, I competed internationally at the Maccabiah Games and won a Bronze medal in a multi-sport Maccabiah Man and Woman competition.

Advice for new vegans?

Don't get overwhelmed -- take it one day at a time. It takes time to get used to any new diet.

Favorite restaurant/recipe?

Vinh Loi Tofu, CA
My Green Smoothie Recipe: 3/4 cup almond milk, kale, carrots, celery, banana, and serving of Sun Warrior protein powder.

Check out Dr. Shenkman's new book, *The Vegan Heart Doctor's Guide to Reversing Heart Disease, Losing Weight, and Reclaiming Your Life***!!**

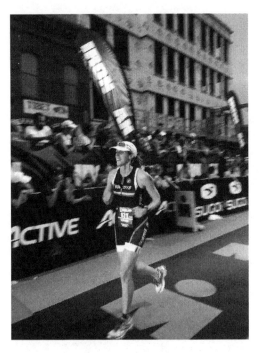

Dr. Heather Shenkman running an Iron Man, Boulder CO, 2005. Photo courtesy of Dr. Shenkman

LEON JACKSON

Staff Sergeant in the New Jersey Air National Guard

How long have you been vegan?

I went vegan on my 22ⁿᵈ birthday, February 9ᵗʰ 2013.

How/why did you go vegan and why are you still vegan?

To be honest, I went vegan because I decided that it was time for a change. I've always been super active and sports played a major role in my life. I was at the point where I thought I was in the best physical shape of my life, but at the same time my body was failing me. I was always in constant pain fighting off tendonitis, so I was constantly searching for ways to restore my body. I firmly believe that food is the natural medicine, so I started there. That's when I discovered that milk/ casein protein was a huge contributor to inflammation. I was really surprised by that, but it all began to make sense! I was taking a ton of whey and casein protein as well as ordering extra cheese on my omelets, which is why my tendons were inflaming. So that's when I became a little more conscious about what exactly entered my body. But it wasn't until I discovered Kathy Freston's book, *The Veganist*, that I decided to give veganism a shot. Every day I feel like I grow and become molded by veganism. I become more passionate about our planet, the animals we share earth with and humanity. These are the structures that I believe in and this is why I remain vegan.

How has being vegan changed your life?

I think it's important that we do something in our lifetime that directly gives back to our children, our community and the

191

earth. Being vegan has influenced me to be more conscious and accountable of my actions. Being vegan has inspired me to go green and to become more compassionate towards all things living.

Tell me about something cool that you've done.

I've been lucky enough to put together a really cool community. It all started when I created an Instagram account (@Vegan_Jiu_Jitsu). From there I was able to connect with a group of vegans who also train in various martial arts, mainly Brazilian Jiu Jitsu. We all share similar interests but different stories. My goal was to show that vegans aren't what society makes us out to be. We come in all different shapes and sizes, and frankly a lot of us kick butt! I created a symbol that represents all Vegan Jiu Jitsu practitioners and a website as well as social media sites where we can tell our own personal stories! I've been receiving a ton of support and I really feel like this is an awesome way to show that "anything you can do; I can do vegan". For more information about us, check out at VeganJiuJitsu.com!

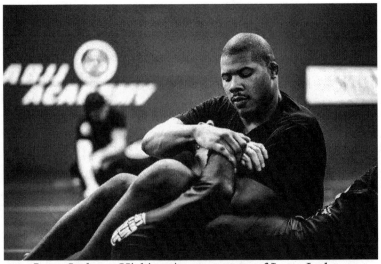

Leon Jackson Kicking Ass, courtesy of Leon Jackson.

Advice for new vegans?

I would suggest to any new vegan that you take the time to do some research. I've seen a lot of people fail because of poor diets (i.e. eating a pack of Oreos every day). We live in a society which enables everyone to have access to instant information. Find someone who can coach you or just answer questions to from time to time. Also remember why you started in the first place and use that as your motivation every day.

Favorite restaurant?

I could never name one place as my favorite, but I do frequent a few restaurants in the New Jersey/Philly area. To name a few, Kaya's Kitchen in Belmar, NJ, The Cinnamon Snail Food Truck in Red Bank, NJ and HipCity Veg, Black Bird Pizzeria, Grindcore House all of which are in Philadelphia.

CORY STANLEY-STAHR

Bee Biologist/Ecologist

How long have you been vegan?

I have been vegan since 2001.

How/why did you go vegan and why are you still vegan?

I became a lacto-ovo vegetarian because I was concerned about animal welfare and also just didn't feel comfortable eating the flesh of another living creature. However, I was not ready to make the move to veganism for a while, mostly because I didn't understand how to cook vegan food and still be healthy. Eventually, I just couldn't conscionably continue consuming eggs and dairy products, knowing the types of cruelty that occur in those industries. Plus, I just felt that, if I can survive without consuming animal products, then why not be vegan? I don't eat humans or drink human breast milk, and in my mind there is not much difference between species. I guess that has always been an issue in my mind as well — speciesism. Why is it OK to eat certain species but not others? I'm not suggesting cannibalism. I'm questioning the ethics behind segregating animals into groups such as pets, livestock, pests, etc. All animals deserve respect.

I continue to be vegan because I can. I have learned how to prepare affordable, nutritious vegan food. The increasing number of vegan foods on the market helps a lot. I have been asked many times, if I were to raise my own chickens, which I'm considering, would I eat their eggs, knowing that the chickens were well-cared for. I don't think I could. I just don't see why I would want to when there are other options.

How has being vegan changed your life?

Being vegan influences my life in several ways. Some are more mundane, such as influencing my choice of restaurant or shampoo. But on a larger scale, being vegan has made me more aware of the world around me. I am more environmentally conscious, because learning about animal welfare has also led me to learn about other issues impacting our world. Also, I just feel like I can more easily see the beauty in the world. I can see the intrinsic beauty of every animal, even the insects, and every plant, even the so-called weeds, more readily because I appreciate their value.

Being vegan also influenced my career choice. I went to school knowing I wanted to be a scientist, and I gravitated toward the life sciences. However, I was dismayed to see how some scientists would recognize how wonderful a particular animal is and seem compelled to cut it up and see how it worked. That was definitely not for me. However, I could see the obvious dependence that man has on bees, and how we are inextricably tied to them because of their pollination services. I love learning about them and about how we can be supportive of them. It is nice to do something positive and not just take from the world, but learn how to give back. I would be lying if I said bees never die in the course of my research, but I hope that in the end, more will live than if I hadn't done the research at all.

Tell me about something cool that you've done.

I started my adult life as a homeless drug addict and eventually became a self-sustaining Ph.D. Biologist who gives back to the community. I have worked with many charities, including a wild bird rehabilitation center, a dog rescue, and a volunteer tax service for low income folks. Currently I am helping the government officials in my town to create a community garden.

Advice for new vegans?

Get out of your "cooking comfort zone." The more you see that vegan food can be prepared easily and economically, the more likely you'll be successful. At first I was really dependent on meat substitutes, but now I don't have to depend on them so much because I can cook tofu, tempeh, and beans. I use the phone app "yummly" a lot. They also have a website, www.yummly.com. You can set it so that it only finds vegan recipes, and it searches metadata, meaning it will search other websites to find a ton of recipe options. Most of them are pretty straightforward and don't require special skills or ingredients.

Favorite recipe/ restaurant?

I have so many favorite recipes. One of the first things I veganized was a recipe for sweet potato casserole. My whole family begs me to make it for family gatherings. I usually double the recipe for the topping, because that's the yummiest part.

Sweet Potato Casserole

Serves 15-20
Base:
- ▶ 3 c. mashed cooked sweet potatoes
- ▶ 7.5 oz. or about 1 cup melted Earth Balance margarine
- ▶ 1 c. vegan granulated sugar
- ▶ Ener-G egg replacer plus water to equal 3 eggs
- ▶ 1 tsp. vanilla
- ▶ ½ c. almond milk (or whatever your favorite vegan milk is)
- ▶ ½ c. self-rising flour (not plain flour)
- ▶ Mix ingredients with mixer. Put in a casserole dish (9x13) and sprinkle with topping. Bake at 350° for 30 minutes.

Topping:
- ► ½ c. brown sugar
- ► ¼ c. Earth Balance margarine
- ► ¼ c. self-rising flour
- ► ½ c. pecans

Mix dry ingredients. Cut in margarine. Sprinkle on sweet potato mixture.

MARY RITA FOSTER

Marketing Specialist

How long have you been vegan?

Vegetarian for 29 years, Vegan since 2007.

How/why did you go vegan and why are you still vegan?

I became a vegetarian as a child when I made the connection that my food was once alive. My father was a hunter and it was quite the journey. I gave up eggs in college, after studying the gestation periods of chickens. At 31, I learned that the veal industry existed because of the dairy industry. I went cold turkey that same day.

I am still vegan because it still matters. I knew it would be a life-long endeavor for me. I felt such a spiritual awakening after I made the change. I can't imagine ever going back. I've also stayed vegan because of all the resources out there: vegan communities, readily available foods, vegan-friendly restaurants, great apps like Happy Cow. Additionally, my partner at the time of my transition was extremely supportive. When he came home from work that day, I explained my feelings and he drove me straight to the book store for vegan cookbooks and nutritional information. We learned how to cook vegan together. I couldn't have made such a graceful transition without him!

How has being vegan changed your life?

Shortly after becoming vegan, I linked up with other members of the vegan community. I attended events and it brought me closer to others who understood how I felt. I also started working for a vegan nutritional resource company. My choice to go vegan has become a way of life, and after the first few weeks it's been more or less a no brainer.

Tell me about something cool that you've done.

I attended a veggie prom, a veggie pride parade, and ran on a vegan running team

Advice for new vegans?

It's so much more than just lettuce -- the internet is your best friend! Learn about nutrition. I read *Vegetarian Cooking for Dummies* and *Becoming Vegan*. Link up with the American Vegan Society. Join vegan potlucks via meetup.com. The people there will teach you yummy recipes, like Alfredo sauce & manicotti. The possibilities are limitless! You can also check out recipes on VegWeb.com

Favorite restaurants?

Vegan Cinnabuns (yep! just like the place in the mall) via VegWeb.com, Vedge & V Street, both in Philadelphia.

LUKE MUIR

LA Area Police Officer

How long have you been vegan?

I have been vegan since my 17th birthday, in 1993.

Why did you go vegan?

I was into punk rock music and going to shows with friends. Vegetarianism was big in the scene. There were a lot of PETA dudes at the shows handing out flyers. I went vegetarian at age 16 and vegan on my 17th birthday. The author of this book is my brother and he was an inspiration as well.

How has being vegan changed your life?

I would say this: it certainly hasn't made things easy. I've always worked blue collar jobs, from construction to tow truck driver to policeman, and not many co-workers in those fields share my beliefs about not eating meat. There isn't a day that goes by that there isn't some ball-breakery. They are even more confused when I explain that I'm doing this for the animals and not for health reasons. Yet, besides all of the jokes, most of my co-workers and friends have been tolerant and try some of my vegan restaurants. Even one of my bosses who is an avid hunter will bring into work vegan desserts that his wife's friend makes from time to time. I'm now living in the LA area so veganism is more commonplace. Every restaurant has a vegan option. When I went vegan in 1993, I would just bake tofu and eat that. My goodness, we have come a long way. For the most part, you can get just about anything you need at a regular supermarket and not have to go to the local health food store to eat vegan.

If you asked my wife how veganism has changed me, she would probably tell you that I've become food obsessed. I have a sweet tooth. I'll make it a mission (or an adventure) to find vegan sweets. Candy/donuts/whatever. However, I've also made sure that I stay in good shape by exercising and eating right. It is possible to get the calcium and protein that you need without eating meat or consuming dairy.

Tell me about something cool that you've done.

In 2005 I completed a thru-hike of the Appalachian Trail. The AT (as it is known) is a 2175 mile hiking trail that runs from Georgia to Maine. It was certainly more of a mental accomplishment than a physical one, but it did take a toll on my body. I started at 205 lbs. and ended at 175 lbs. My main diet at that time was dried fruit and nuts for a snack and PBJ for lunch and TVP and elbow macaroni for dinner. The hike lasted 4 months and 20 days. It was a beautiful walk with plenty of time for reflection.

Advice for new vegans?

Don't get carried away. When I was in my late teens/early 20s I thought that it was important to be super strict with myself. I remember going to a local Chinese restaurant and ordering Bean Curd Szechwan. After I had started eating I realized that there was something weird about the bean curd, so I asked the lady who worked there and she and she told me that it was chicken. I went to the drug store and bought ipecac to make me vomit the meat out because I thought that was the right thing to do. If you get too carried away with anything its hard to maintain. I don't think that I would still be vegan if I got upset anytime I accidentally ate something that I didn't intend to eat. I could never go out to eat, and I could never eat at my parent's house if I was that overly concerned about cross contamination.

I think this can be a healthy diet, but just because something doesn't contain animal doesn't make it healthy. Potato chips and soda can be vegan, but of course they are not good for you. That being said, too much tofu isn't good for you either. My dad, who is much smarter than I am, always says that moderation is the key. For new vegans, the 3 essentials are: 1. Eat right. 2. Enjoy what you are eating 3. Don't get too stressed out about the little stuff. For example, I was friends with a vegan guy who told me that he wouldn't chew Big Red gum because he heard that Red Dye #5 (an ingredient in Big Red) is made of crushed lady bugs. That guy isn't vegan, or even vegetarian, anymore.

Favorite Restaurants?

I'm not much of a cook. I can make tacos with Boca crumbles, spaghetti, and maybe toast. My wife is a good cook, and she makes her own seitan. I can't really give one favorite restaurant, so I'll have to give you my list: I'm from Philadelphia, and the best place to get a Pizza or Cheesesteaks is Blackbird Pizza. My friend Mark owns this pizzeria and has perfected the Vegan Philly cheesesteak. As far as fancy sit down restaurants go, Vedge in Philadelphia is the top of the mountain. There are a ton of vegan Thai places in LA that are good. There is a chain of restaurants called "Veggie Grill" that has a lot of good stuff. Something that I just discovered for anyone who goes to Las Vegas is every restaurant at the Wynn Hotel has a vegan option now, including French toast and milkshakes.

LYNN ANN DE FRANCESCO RISOR

Payroll processor

How long have you been vegan?

I have been vegan since June of 2011

How/why did you go vegan and why are you still vegan?

I was attempting to lose weight and knew something was going on. My family has a history of diabetes so that was my fear. I made an appointment with my GYN. He did an extensive blood test and sure enough I was a type II diabetic. Fortunately for me, my doctor followed John McDougall, MD, so he prompted me to try what he called an "extreme vegan diet" for one week. The alternative was prescribing medication. I did not want to get diabetes, as I have seen family members go through this, even having one die due to complications of the disease. So for one week I tried and struggled, but for me the catalyst for me was the weight loss I experienced in just one week's time. I lost quite a bit of weight the first 6 months I was vegan, 50lbs in all. Now almost four years later I am still vegan, but have put some of the weight back on simply because of stated bad behaviors. I stay vegan first and foremost because I do not want to sink back into diabetes again. I am also vegan because I have been exposed to the cruelty and harm that is done to animals in the factory farming industry. I remember seeing feedlot cattle standing in their own urine and feces and thinking about how unhappy they looked. I didn't even know the half of it back then, and that the truth was far worse than I thought. And it's not just the meat/dairy/fishing industry, but also the clothing, cosmetic and pharmaceutical industries as well that use animals in other practices other than eating. That is why I stay vegan.

How has being vegan changed your life?

It definitely has changed my circle of friends. I have a few friends who really take the time to make sure there is something I can eat if invited. With others it's really fend for yourself. The vegan crowd is a much smaller one, but it's growing, thank goodness! And I have had the pleasure of meeting some pretty amazing people along the way. Definitely a much different crowd than I used to be around. It also influences the types of activities you participate in, such as NOT going to a zoo, aquarium, or aquatic park such as Sea World. I realized these are not places these creatures need to be, nor do children need these places to "learn" about animals and sea creatures. Being vegan also made me much more aware of the health of my own body and how food affects it, even though I am still overweight and struggling to get a handle on that. My blood tests always come out really clean. I have good cholesterol levels, good vitamin levels, great protein levels and no diabetes, no high blood pressure, no heart problems. Also so far, I have no signs of cancer which also seems pretty prevalent in my family. Wanting good health has also influenced me to get out and move more. One has to exercise everyday even if it's simply taking a brisk walk a couple of times around the block! My dream is to one day open up a vegan B&B somewhere close to the beach, with a small side café. I think I'd be really good at that!

Tell me about something cool that you've done.

One of the coolest things I have done while vegan is complete in what is called the "Warrior Dash." I wasn't shooting for a prize, but just to finish it. It's a 5K run through a boot camp type obstacle trail in the mountains in Edgewood, NM. It was very cool (and cold). I was 49 years old at the time, and with little training I actually dealt with some fears and finished in 1 hour and 10 minutes, while my 29-year-old daughter did it in an hour. I felt pretty darn good about being only 10 minutes slower than someone 20 years younger!! The biggest accomplishment for me in that obstacle course was the cargo net at the finish line. Being afraid of heights I took one look at that, about 20ft high, and said internally, "no f'n way" and then proceeded to climb over it to the other side. Even my husband was impressed. It was a good day!

Advice for new vegans?

Make sure you learn about what is happening to the animals used for food, furniture, shoes, and testing so that you can be aware. Being "connected" help keeps you vegan and compassionate. Learn what factory farming is doing to our planet; it's being destroyed rather quickly. Don't be afraid to try new things. Use the Internet as a tool; there are so many good recipes / blogs / and tips out there it will blow your mind. Stick to whole-foods as much as possible, and try to stay away from the processed foods. If you must have something like the sausages or meatballs, learn how to make them yourself so YOU know the ingredients! They are much simpler than you think. Get involved in vegan meet up groups so you will be with like minded people. There is power in numbers and friendships!

Favorite recipe/ restaurant?

There is simply more than one recipe. I am one who loves to cook, and my favorite dishes lean towards Italian, Hispanic and Indian dishes. They seem to have the most flavor and very easy to make vegan, especially the Indian curries. I love to make breads, quick breads and artisan breads. If must pick one dish that I love to make it would be lasagna.

My favorite restaurants would be Thai Vegan in Albuquerque, New Mexico, and in Gainesville Florida it is without a doubt Gyro's Plus, oh my goodness they rock.

David Risor

Carpenter

How long have you been vegan?

I have been vegan since 2011.

How/why did you go vegan and why are you still vegan?

Besides being a vegan redneck (which is rare), I call myself an accidental vegan. My wife had diabetes, and the doctor recommended a vegan diet. I had all intentions of only going pescetarian. After a few weeks, the eggs and cheese ran out, the food was decent, and my wife was seeing results. I said what the hell and started doing the vegan thing along with her.

How has being vegan changed your life?

Being vegan started with health, however I have come to focus on environmental issues and animal welfare as well. Becoming vegan improved my joint health, and helped me drop almost 50 lbs. I started up running again, soon became a running addict, and now run around 40 miles a week even in the off season. As a side note, my father was a butcher, so as the vegan son of a butcher, my life is somewhat amusing.

Tell me about something cool that you've done.

As I said before, I run a lot. Mountain trails have been a large part of my running culture. In 2014 I won a position for the La Luz trail run, one of my favorite trails, in Albuquerque, New Mexico. There are only 400 runners who are determined by a lottery. It has been ranked as one of the most difficult trail races in the US, due to it's terrain, and has over 6000 feet of elevation gain in 9 miles. And yes, I did complete the run somewhere in mid pack. I also managed to run a 10k during which I beat out most of a high school track team, finishing 6th place overall and 1st in my age group.

Advice for new vegans?

There is a lot of advice out there, some good and some bad. Don't listen to every extreme thing you hear. You will eventually find what works for you and your body.

Favorite recipe/ restaurant?

My favorite recipe varies, somewhere between black bean burgers and jackfruit tacos. Favorite restaurant – probably Thai Vegan on Osuna in Albuquerque, NM.

JOYCE DiBENEDETTO-COLTON

Retired educator

How long have you been vegan?

Since about 1996. Became vegetarian in 1975. Then, influenced by relationship changes, consumed some fish and poultry for a time, then once again returned to a vegetarian diet until 1996, when animal products were eliminated from my diet completely.

How/why did you go vegan and why are you still vegan?

I was vegetarian predominantly for health reasons. Over the years it became more of an ethical issue. Choosing to go vegan was for multiple reasons: to maximize my health, to help prevent animal suffering, to reduce my environmental impact, as well as to affect the market/economy — I didn't want to subsidize companies that negatively impacted our world.

How has being vegan changed your life?

This is not a simple question to answer. A vegan lifestyle aligns with my beliefs. Being a vegan has allowed me to find meaningful relationships with other veg people, but it has, more often than I'd like, caused a sense of judgementalism on the part of non-vegans and vegans alike. As I get older, I'm more content to do my own thing and don't concern myself with the views of others regarding what I eat. In other ways, because being vegan is not mainstream, it is considerably more of a challenge. We vegans are always having to "watch" for insidious ingredients in foods, or be cognizant of avoiding cruelties practiced by companies. And what's with the "vegetarian" sections on restaurant menus?? Most of the items are full of cheese. How patronizing is that? If restaurant owners were actually aware, they would have "vegan" menu sections, and let vegetarians add cheese if they need to. How about that!? (I say this in a comedic – but sorrowful way.)

Tell me about something cool that you've done.

By this point in my life I can say there have been lots of "cool" things I've done. Some of the most rewarding have been preparing great vegan food for events – even when the event was not a "vegan" one. In the college where I worked I was able to organize many events to educate students, faculty, and staff about food choices.

Advice for new vegans?

Eat whole organic foods. Always carry a Ziploc with raw almonds and dried fruit in your bag.

Favorite recipe/ restaurant?

Sorry – my fav dish is still mixed organic salad. I love Thai food. I'm not big on restaurants, but when we go out, we usually choose Asian. I also like East Indian dishes (that I prepare.) And I'm Italian, so pasta, polenta, risotto – all with lots of veggies and herbs! …Hey! – I'm-a gettin' hungry here!

Rob Beaton

Food Service Director for Upper Columbia Academy,
a vegetarian cafe

How long have you been vegan?

I have been vegan since 1994

How/why did you go vegan and why are you still vegan?

Studying with the Seventh Day Adventist Church, I realized that my body was Jesus's Temple and he wanted to be resurrected through me, so that my hands, feet, mouth, words, eyes, ears, and even my very thoughts could be His. In order for this to happen, I needed to keep my body as pure as I could by abstaining from all pollutants such as alcohol, nicotine, drugs of any types, meat and meat by products. This would help my blood to be free of the miasma that would cloud my mind that would retard my ability to commune with God through prayer and the study of His Word.

How has being vegan changed your life?

It affects where I work, the friends that I have, and the relationships I'm in. I pray that Jesus through me has had an influence over young people that will give them a better quality of life. But my prayer is not just to live longer on a dying planet, but also to live forever with Him who gave me this message, and to train my taste buds for heavenly food. Up in heaven a chicken will be totally uninhibited to walk right in front of me without fear that I will snatch her up, break her neck and roast her over a fire, and slap him between two slices of bread and eat him, nor her unborn fetus! I will be able to watch him walk in front of me without drool running down my face.

Tell me about something cool that you've done.

In 2005 there was a large vegetarian convention that was happening in Cincinnati, Ohio, that Chef Tupolo and I were invited to consult with. This was a very difficult thing to do. Most Chefs will not accept advice from a "consultant," because that would mean that they had to admit that they didn't know everything about food. Chef Tupolo and I created a breakfast tofu with turmeric, garlic, onions, McKay's Vegan Chicken seasoning, Braggs aminos nutritional yeast etc. for about 2500 people. The chefs in the back of the kitchen were stunned. They thought it tasted almost like scrambled eggs. They stated that the texture was a little different but the flavor was incredible.

Advice for new vegans?

People who are changing over to this type of eating need to realize that their taste buds are perverted by eating the S.A.D. diet, or by eating the S.O.S diet, which is too much Salt, Oil, & Sugar. I would recommend a minimum of a 3- day fast before beginning a total vegan diet; even a 7- day fast would not hurt. I do advocate a complete and immediate switch over. I would not recommend a slow change. I believe that could be recipe for failure. There are a lot of meat analogs out there and meat substitutes, some of them are quite tasty. I would steer away from these as a lot of them are more difficult to digest by the body than is meat! My personal conviction on most food is that the closer you can eat it to the way God made it, the better off you are. When selecting an almond to eat, no need to roast it, season it, dip it in chocolate. Get used to eating a raw almond, which is really the best for you. Our food should be our medicine, but unlike a lot of medicine, we should not have to pinch our nose and swallow it quickly with a shot of water to chase it down. Our food should look good, taste good, and be good for us, and not necessarily in that order either.

Favorite recipe/ restaurant?

I am a baker, and have lately been dabbling in sprouted, flourless whole wheat bread. When one gets the right wheat, one can sprout it for about 24 to 36 hours and then run it through a meat grinder (the best use for a meat grinder) then just add salt and yeast, proof it, bake it, slice it, and you have a terrific tasting loaf of bread. I have discovered that the more I work in the restaurant business, the more I like to eat at home. Lots of nasty things happen out there and very poor personal hygiene is happening in restaurants today. But If I have to pick one it would be P.F. Chang's Tofu-coconut curry plate.

JESSICA TRUE

Promotional model/Brand ambassador

How long have you been vegan?

I turned vegetarian when I was 15 or 16, and I kept learning more and more about how awful the egg and dairy industries are, so I made a gradual switch to vegan through the end of high school and beginning of college. I have been vegan since 2012 and have never felt better.

How/why did you go vegan and why are you still vegan?

I turned vegan for the animals initially, and I'm staying vegan for the animals and for the health benefits. I grew up eating McDonalds weekly and I come from a family with many health issues that I don't exactly wish to partake in. This is me trying my very best to avoid them and set a better example for my family. I know I've already influenced many of their eating decisions.

How has being vegan changed your life?

Being vegan has completely influenced my life. It isn't just a diet; it's a lifestyle. My boyfriend of 5 years is vegetarian and he eats a lot of vegan food with me. I know if he didn't have the same mindset about something so important to me that we wouldn't have made it so far. Finding new vegan restaurants is one of our favorite things to do. Being vegan has also made me want to have my own vegan road trips and have a better, cleaner impact on the world. My future plans also include opening a sanctuary for rescued factory farm animals, and hopefully opening a vegan restaurant at some point. Delicious vegan food makes me giddy, and I want to share that with everyone.

Tell me about something cool that you've done.

I've influenced a lot of friends and family to turn vegetarian (it's a start!) and I also fell in love with a chicken at a local petting zoo years ago. The goats in the zoo were walking around trying to eat the fur on the rabbits and the feathers on the chickens, so she climbed up into my lap and trusted me. Just thinking back to that moment years ago reminds me that animals are here with feelings and emotions and the ability to love and trust, just as we are. Just because they don't speak my language doesn't mean we don't speak the same feelings.

Advice for new vegans?

Take baby steps, and don't limit yourself. Try new foods; there are so many cultures full of vegan foods with exhilarating new flavors that you have yet to try. My motto is, if I can eat it, I will. I will not fear a new vegetable or fruit or dish, because being vegan truly is limitless, especially with all the new substitutes out there to help you along the way. There's also a super tight-knit vegan community on social media and in all big cities. I've met vegans in California and England just with the use of that beautiful little #vegan. Good luck!

Favorite recipe?

My favorite recipes are constantly changing. I think one that won't be changing is from the vegan food blog *Oh She Glows*. Angela at *Oh She Glows* is a vegan wizard, and I'm in love with her Quick and Dirty 5-Ingredient Vegan Cheeze Sauce. I've made my own adaptations through the years and I've also learned to love nutritional yeast (also lovingly referred to by many as Nooch).

Favorite restaurant?

My favorite vegan restaurant is also always changing, but right now my boyfriend and I have become very fond of a tiny 17-seat restaurant in Chicago called Kitchen 17. Don, the owner and chef, is also a vegan wizard. He is constantly changing the menu, adapting dishes to the preferences of individual diners, making things that aren't even on the menu, and right now, he has a line of foods which he markets with #irrationallyvegan. This line includes vegan deep dish pizza, one of the foods that Chicago is most well-known for, calzones, milkshakes, sausage gravy and biscuits, fettuccini alfredo, and vegan beef stroganoff. Just thinking of the menu is making me so hungry right now!

GEORGE MCQUADE

U.S. Army Medic, (68W, 68L, 68X)
Purple Hearts and Minds cofounder and activist

How long have you been vegan?

Since January 2005.

How/why did you go vegan?

I was on my second deployment to Iraq with a psychologist who is vegan as my Officer in Charge. I began to ask all of the typical questions that people ask vegans and began to do my own research as well. I soon realized that there was no need to cause harm at this scale to animals. There was an alternative. I learned of the impact that Animal Agriculture has on the environment and the adverse health effects directly linked to consumption of animal products. The only reason not to change would be my own selfishness and blatant disregard for all life on the plant to include my own. Vegan is the present; if you aren't vegan, you are living in the past. If we don't act now, there won't be a future.

How does being vegan affect your life/influence the directions that your life has gone in?

I have become a much more compassionate person and am much more aware of how my decisions in consumption and lifestyle have a direct impact on the lives of others. I am much more concerned with health and fitness, where my food comes from and producing food. Living with minimal waste and as local as possible is something I value much more. Being vegan has brought me closer to other vegans and brought me to the realization that we can all use better self-care and make a difference in this world. I am currently working on different approaches in activism as well as a resiliency group and resources for activists. After over a decade in activism in several parts of the country, it became apparent at how much more support vegans and activists need. This goes from self-care, to gaining insight, improving communication, conflict resolution, non-violence training, to simply setting the example to others who are interested in learning about living vegan. I also have a nonprofit with another veteran focused on nonviolence. It is both an avenue to living with compassion as a vegan with minimal impact and a safe environment for healing and growth for those who are struggling after transitioning from the military. There are a few other projects that I am working on that will continue to develop over the coming months.

Any advice for vegans interested in activism?

As discussed before, self-care is everything. Success does not come from exhausted yourself, rather it is a result of a balanced healthy life and an alignment with your own values and passion. Learn everything you can and reach out to others who can help. Spread the love so that we can all live in better place. Ahimsa

Favorite recipe/other restaurant?

Millennium in Oakland is still my favorite restaurant because I went there for the first time with my girlfriend for her birthday. Check out her developing business, Ellora Wellness on Instagram, Facebook, Twitter, or www.ellorawellness.com. As far as recipes, I really have so many things that I enjoy. There is a common misperception that being vegan is restrictive because of the prevalence of carnism and mass marketing leading people to believe that animals are necessary for development and survival. When we are out in environments where the focus is animal remains on a plate, we end up with items being taken off a plate. The end result seems to be an iceberg lettuce salad with shredded carrots and oil and vinegar dressing. The plate which contained the standard American diet items originally has been reduced to steamed broccoli and if you are lucky, a baked potato. Vegans certainly don't want the flesh of a cow or their secretions in the mashed potatoes. The point is, being vegan will without a doubt expand your offerings. The perspective must be on how we enrich our lives with compassionate choices and items we haven't taken the opportunity to be familiar. Ethnic restaurants and fare is so diverse and rewarding to discover. Sharing vegan items from different cultures is a rewarding aspect of socializing as a vegan. Everyone has eaten vegan before and often doesn't realize it. Living vegan is the only way for us to continue else we accept our fate in a similar parallel to those who are crying and ignored to those not yet ready to accept the reality of the animal holocaust.

OUTRO

I STARTED WRITING *VEGAN STRONG* in 2014 as a response to the meat-eaters around me who believed a person couldn't be strong without eating meat. As a longtime vegan and former US ARMY Paratrooper, marathon runner, and martial artist, I felt the need to speak out against this misconception. While I believe this book, along with other excellent books such as *The China Study* and *How Not to Die* successfully refute those outdated views of nutrition, I feel my reason for writing *VEGAN STRONG* has changed along the journey. Allow me to explain.

I am not proud of this book simply because it is a statement <u>against</u> eating meat. You can get that message anywhere. Hell, Morrissey has been singing "Meat is Murder" since 1985. Instead, I am proud of this book because it is my statement of <u>life</u> in these troubled times. I became a vegan during my punk rock years because I wanted to save the world, and have remained vegan all these years because it a lifestyle that has been proved time and again to be the healthiest way of living -- for me, for the animals, and for the planet. My love of life is the strength of this book, and that positivity is what I am proud to have shared with you in *VEGAN STRONG*.

Well, there you have it folks. We have explored the ins and outs of the cultural phenomenon of veganism. We have talked about the importance of being vegan from environmental, health, and compassion standpoints. We have learned about nutrition, what to eat and what not to eat, and why, and have heard from a variety of voices on the topic. I hope that you have also learned how to cook some delicious vegan dishes and are even more excited to work out. Whether this book has helped you to become vegan or just eat a little healthier, my sincere hope is that you have enjoyed yourself along the way. Thanks for reading.

-SGT Vegan
(Bill Muir, RN. BSN)

REFERENCES

Part 1: VEGAN STRONG

1. Crowe, F.L., Appleby, P. N., Travis, R.C., Key, T.J., Risk of hospitalization or death from ischemic heart disease among British vegetarians and non-vegetarians: results from the EPIC-Oxford cohort study. The American Journal of Clinical Nutrition, January 30, 2013, doi:10.3945/ajcn.112.044073

2. Position of American Dietetic Association on Vegetarian Diet: J Am Diet Assoc. 2009 Jul;109(7):1266-82

3. Greger, Michael, M.D. How Not To Die, Flatiron Books,2015 (pg 53)

4. Crowe, F.L., Appleby, P. N., Travis, R.C., Key, T.J., Risk of hospitalization or death from ischemic heart disease among British vegetarians and non-vegetarians: results from the EPIC-Oxford cohort study. The American Journal of Clinical Nutrition, January 30, 2013, doi:10.3945/ajcn.112.044073

5. Campbell, T. Colin, PhD, The China Study, Benbella Books, Inc. 2006 (pg117)

6. Greger, Michael, M.D. How Not To Die, Flatiron Books,2015 (pg 124-125)

7. Greger, Michael, M.D. How Not To Die, Flatiron Books,2015 (pg 347-348)

8. Campbell, T. Colin, PhD, The China Study, Benbella Books, Inc. 2006 (pg 139)

9. Simon, Stacy. World Health Organization Says Processed Meat Causes Cancer Article date: October 26, 2015 American Cancer Society- cancer.org

10. Campbell, T. Colin, PhD, The China Study, Benbella Books, Inc. 2006 (pg 151)

11. Campbell, T. Colin, PhD, The China Study, Benbella Books, Inc. 2006 (pg 152)

12. www.cowspiracy.com, "The Facts, " toward the bottom of the page

13. Alman, Ashley. Al Gore Goes Vegan. The Huffington Post. Posted 11/25/2013 huffingtonpost.com

14. Al Gore interview- Lateline ABC, Broadcast 04/11/2009 abc.net.au

15. Steinfield, Henning, et all. Livestock's Long Shadow: Environmental Issues and Options. Food and Agriculture Organization of the United Nations. Rome 2006 (pg 272)

16. Goodland, Robert & Anhang, Jeff. "Livestock and Climate Change: What if the key actors in climate change are...cows, pigs and chickens?". WorldWatch. November/December 2009. Worldwatch.org (pg 11)

17. Before Trump era control of the United States Government, the EPA had this on their website, www3.epa.gov "Livestock, especially cattle, produce methane ($CH4$) as part of their digestion. This process is called enteric fermentation, and it represents almost one third of the emissions from the Agriculture sector. The way in which manure from livestock is managed also contributes to $CH4$ and $N2O$ emissions. Manure storage methods and the amount of exposure to oxygen and moisture can affect how these greenhouse gases are produced. Manure management accounts for about 14% of the total greenhouse gas emissions from the Agriculture sector in the United States."

18. Lundqvist, J.,C. de Fraiture, D. Molden. Saving Water: From Field to Fork – Curbing Losses and Wastage in the Food Chain. SIWI Policy Brief. SIWI, 2008 (pg11)

19. Pimentel, David, et all., Ecological Integrity: Integrating Environment, Conservation, and Health. Island Press, 2000 (pg 129).

20. Walsh, Bryan. The Triple Whopper Environmental Impact of Global Meat Production. Time. (science.time.com) Dec 16, 2013

21. Environmental Protection Agency. Water Quality Conditions in the United States-A Profile from the 2000 National Water Quality Inventory www.epa.gov (pg 1)

22. Steinfield, Henning, et all. Livestock's Long Shadow: Environmental Issues and Options. Food and Agriculture Organization of the United Nations. Rome 2006 (pg 270)

23. "Happy Cows, Behind the Myth", humanemyth.org

24. McWilliams, James. "Milk of Human Kindness denied to Dairy Cows." Forbes.com, Oct 25, 2013

25. Stein, Rob. "Study: More milk means more weight gain." Washington Post. June 7, 2005

26. "Dairy Fact Sheet"(pg 2), Physicians Committee for Responsible Medicine, www.pcrm.org

27. "Protecting Your Bones". Physicians Committee for Responsible Medicine, www.pcrm.org

28. "Preventing and Reversing Osteoporosis." Physicians Committee for Responsible Medicine, www.pcrm.org

29. 4. Djoussé L, Gaziano JM. "Egg consumption in relation to cardiovascular disease and mortality: the Physicians' Health Study." American Journal of Clinical Nutrition, April 2008.

30. Barnard, Neil, MD FACC, The Cheese Trap: How Breaking a Surprising Addiction Will Help You Lose Weight, Gain Energy, and Get Healthy, 2017 (pg 39-40)

Part 2: VEGAN POWER

31. Patricia Deuster, PHD et all The US Navy Seal Guide to Fitness and Nutrition, Skyhorse Publishing, Inc, 2007. (pg. 291)

32. Patricia Deuster, PHD et all The US Navy Seal Guide to Fitness and Nutrition, Skyhorse Publishing, Inc, 2007. (pg. 293)

33. Patricia Deuster, PHD et all The US Navy Seal Guide to Fitness and Nutrition, Skyhorse Publishing, Inc, 2007. (pg. 290)

34. Kleinfield, N.R. Just What Killed the Diet Doctor, And What Keeps the Issue Alive? The New York Times, Feb 11, 2004

35. Thompson, Dennis Sugar vs. high-fructose corn syrup: Is one sweetener worse for your health? CBS News, cbsnew.com, June 22, 2015

36. Artificial sweeteners and other sugar substitutes – Mayo Clinic: http://www.mayoclinic.org/healthy-lifestyle/nutrition-and-healthy-eating/in-depth/artificial-sweeteners/art-20046936/-62k

37. Migraines Symptoms and Causes -Mayo Clinic http://www.mayoclinic.org/diseases-conditions/migraine-headache/symptoms-causes/dxc-20202434

38. Greger, Michael, M.D. <u>How Not To Die,</u> Flatiron Books,2015 (pg 206)
39. Phenylketonuria (PKU) Treatments and drugs- Mayo Clinic: http://www.mayoclinic.org/diseases-conditions/phenylketonuria/basics/treatment/con-20026275
40. Campbell, T. Colin, PhD, <u>The China Study</u>, Benbella Books, Inc. 2006 (pg 308)
41. Patricia Deuster, PHD et all <u>The US Navy Seal Guide to Fitness and Nutrition</u>, Skyhorse Publishing, Inc., 2007. (pg. 310)
42. Brenda Davis, RD & Vesanto Melina, MS, RD, <u>Becoming Vegan: The Complete Guide to Adopting a Healthy Planet-Based Diet</u>, Book Publishing Company, 2000 (pg. 141)
43. Brenda Davis, RD & Vesanto Melina, MS, RD, <u>Becoming Vegan: The Complete Guide to Adopting a Healthy Planet-Based Diet</u>, Book Publishing Company, 2000 (pg. 129)
44. Nguyen-Khoa, Dieu-Thu, MD, FACP, <u>Beriberi (Thiamine Deficiency)</u>, Medscape (emedicine.medscape.com), Updated: March 2, 2017
45. Brenda Davis, RD & Vesanto Melina, MS, RD, <u>Becoming Vegan: The Complete Guide to Adopting a Healthy Planet-Based Diet</u>, Book Publishing Company, 2000 (pg. 130)
46. Brenda Davis, RD & Vesanto Melina, MS, RD, <u>Becoming Vegan: The Complete Guide to Adopting a Healthy Planet-Based Diet</u>, Book Publishing Company, 2000 (pg. 130)
47. Brenda Davis, RD & Vesanto Melina, MS, RD, <u>Becoming Vegan: The Complete Guide to Adopting a Healthy Planet-Based Diet</u>, Book Publishing Company, 2000 (pg. 130)
48. Brenda Davis, RD & Vesanto Melina, MS, RD, <u>Becoming Vegan: The Complete Guide to Adopting a Healthy Planet-Based Diet</u>, Book Publishing Company, 2000 (pg. 131)
49. Brenda Davis, RD & Vesanto Melina, MS, RD, <u>Becoming Vegan: The Complete Guide to Adopting a Healthy Planet-Based Diet</u>, Book Publishing Company, 2000 (pg. 122-123)
50. Brenda Davis, RD & Vesanto Melina, MS, RD, <u>Becoming Vegan: The Complete Guide to Adopting a Healthy Planet-Based Diet</u>, Book Publishing Company, 2000 (pg. 140)

51. Brenda Davis, RD & Vesanto Melina, MS, RD, <u>Becoming Vegan: The Complete Guide to Adopting a Healthy Planet-Based Diet</u>, Book Publishing Company, 2000 (pg. 137-139)

52. Brenda Davis, RD & Vesanto Melina, MS, RD, <u>Becoming Vegan: The Complete Guide to Adopting a Healthy Planet-Based Diet</u>, Book Publishing Company, 2000 (pg. 141)

53. Brenda Davis, RD & Vesanto Melina, MS, RD, <u>Becoming Vegan: The Complete Guide to Adopting a Healthy Planet-Based Diet</u>, Book Publishing Company, 2000 (pg. 142)

54. Brenda Davis, RD & Vesanto Melina, MS, RD, <u>Becoming Vegan: The Complete Guide to Adopting a Healthy Planet-Based Diet</u>, Book Publishing Company, 2000 (pg.95)

55. Brenda Davis, RD & Vesanto Melina, MS, RD, <u>Becoming Vegan: The Complete Guide to Adopting a Healthy Planet-Based Diet</u>, Book Publishing Company, 2000 (pg. 116)

56. Brenda Davis, RD & Vesanto Melina, MS, RD, <u>Becoming Vegan: The Complete Guide to Adopting a Healthy Planet-Based Diet</u>, Book Publishing Company, 2000 (pg. 105)

57. Brenda Davis, RD & Vesanto Melina, MS, RD, <u>Becoming Vegan: The Complete Guide to Adopting a Healthy Planet-Based Diet</u>, Book Publishing Company, 2000 (pg 118)

58. Brenda Davis, RD & Vesanto Melina, MS, RD, <u>Becoming Vegan: The Complete Guide to Adopting a Healthy Planet-Based Diet</u>, Book Publishing Company, 2000 (pg 119)

59. Brenda Davis, RD & Vesanto Melina, MS, RD, <u>Becoming Vegan: The Complete Guide to Adopting a Healthy Planet-Based Diet</u>, Book Publishing Company, 2000 (pg. 113)

60. Campbell, T. Colin, PhD, <u>The China Study</u>, Benbella Books, Inc. 2006 (pg. 138)

61. Greger, Michael M.D., <u>How Not To Die</u>, Flatiron Books, 2015 (pg.372)

62. Kleinfield, <u>N.R., Just what Killed the Diet Doctor, and What Keeps the Issue Alive</u>, The New York Times, Feb. 11, 2004

63. Haupt, Angela. <u>Ashton Kutcher's Fruitarian Diet: What went wrong</u>? US News & World Report. Feb. 7, 2013

64. Greger, Michael M.D., <u>How Not To Die</u>, Flatiron Books, 2015 (pg.332-333)

65. Greger, Michael M.D., <u>How Not To Die</u>, Flatiron Books, 2015 (pg.334)

66. Greger, Michael M.D., <u>How Not To Die</u>, Flatiron Books, 2015 (pg.333)

52991360R00146

Made in the USA
Lexington, KY
24 September 2019